Advance Pra~~ise f~~
Scott Davi~~s~~
If My Body Is a Temple, The~~n~~

"I have known Scott (and there was a lot of him to know) for many years. Although there is less of him to see now, there is even more of him to love. His story is not only funny but a tender reminder that we must all become healthier inside and out—no matter how much of you there is."

> — **Chonda Pierce, stand-up comic, TV host, and author**

"I've traveled a lot of miles and spent a lot of time with Scott Davis and I've known him as a man who loves Jesus, loves people, and loves, well...food. Now, he's more than 130 pounds thinner and has quite a story to share!"

> — **Mark Hall, lead singer and songwriter, Casting Crowns**

"Most of us wish we could see less of ourselves in the mirror. Scott Davis knows your pain, and then some! This book brings the laughs, but it will also inspire you to follow Scott on the same quest: to seek God's best. And that includes a less-flabby life. Now excuse me, I've got to go brush the cobwebs off of my treadmill."

> — **Cory Edwards, writer/director**
> **of the motion picture "Hoodwinked"**

"I know the 'after' Scott Davis (the guy who wrote this book), and I knew the 'before' Scott Davis (the guy who, by his own admission, might have eaten this book), and they're both hilariously funny guys who have a passion for hurting souls. Scott's story of his journey to a whole new self is going to encourage you, make you laugh, and best of all, it's going to make you think. With Scott's sense of humor ever present, this is the easiest, most painless weight loss book you'll ever digest!"

> — **Martha Bolton, author of more than 50 books and**
> **Emmy-nominated comedy writer on staff with Bob Hope for 15 years**

"Scott Davis seems to have the distinction of being just about everyone's great friend, and that includes me! He is insightful, transparent, and flat-out funny beyond belief, and you will be blessed by his new book, *If My Body Is A Temple, Then I Was A Megachurch*. Scott shares his life-long battle with weight issues and how he gained victory in this crucial area. I think *you* will burn calories laughing your way through the pages of this inspirational masterpiece!"

— **Dr. Dwight "Ike" Reighard, pastor and co-author of**
The One Year Daily Insights with Zig Ziglar

"I saw Scott Davis recently and he's half the man he used to be—literally! As usual, Scott encouraged me, made me laugh, and inspired me to get fit both inside and out. He'll help get you on the right track, too."

— **Babbie Mason, award-winning singer and songwriter**

"Scott Davis has been a good friend of mine for over twenty years and I now have the blessing of serving as his family's pastor. His story is absolutely amazing. Scott's hilarious ability to see life on the lighter-side has kept my life filled with laughter, now he lives on the lighter-side. I can personally testify that he lost his weight with NO exercise but through the diligent discipline of eating the right foods. To be honest, when he began I thought his efforts would prove wasted ... I know how much he loves food! But he wasted no opportunity and now his life is transformed. Today he carries much less weight but his words now carry even more."

— **Tim Dowdy, pastor and author of *Don't Forget to Dream***

If My Body Is a
TEMPLE,
Then I Was a
MEGACHURCH

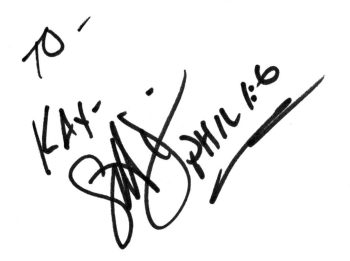

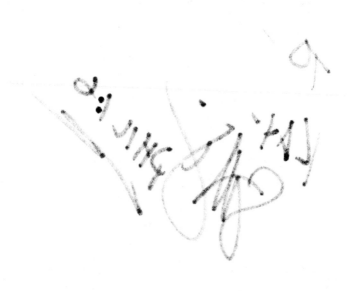

If My Body Is a
TEMPLE,
Then I Was a
MEGACHURCH

Foreword by
Mark Lowry

My journey of losing 132 pounds with no exercise!!

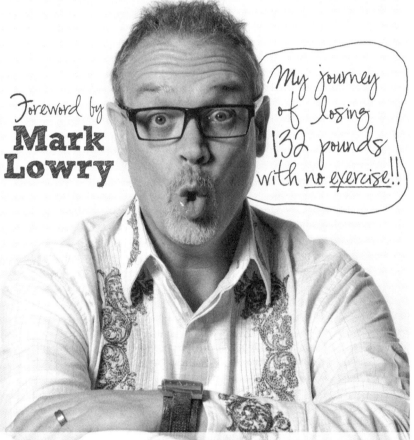

SCOTT DAVIS
WITH TIM LUKE

ampelon PUBLISHING
Boise, ID

ampelōn
pUBLISHING

Ampelon Publishing publishes works that challenge and inspire Christians
to discover the heart of Christ in new and fresh ways

If My Body is a Temple, Then I Was a Megachurch
Copyright ©2011 by Scott Davis

Published by Ampelon Publishing
P.O. Box 140675, Boise, ID 83714
www.AmpelonPublishing.com

Unless otherwise indicated, Bible quotations are taken
from the New King James Version.
Copyright © 1982 by Thomas Nelson, Inc. Used by permission. All rights reserved.

Cover & inside design: Jared Swafford — SwingFromTheRafters.com

ISBN: 978-0-9823286-4-4
Library of Congress Control Number: 2011913060

Printed in the United States of America
on paper made from sustainable resources

To my mother Geneva F. Davis, who went home to Heaven on October 25, 2001

DISCLAIMER

In this book I share my opinions about weight control and health issues and their causes. These opinions are just that—opinions—and they're based on personal experience and knowledge gained from trying various diets and exercises. As my daddy used to say, I ain't no doctor. So don't stake your health or your life on something I say or write.

Consult your physician before trying to diet, lose weight, or exercise, or if you have medical questions. Since I have a nerdy-looking attorney with chic European glasses, slicked-back hair, and a musty tweed jacket staring over my shoulder, I must tell you that I cannot be held responsible for any decisions or weight-loss or exercise attempts you make as a result of reading this book. I repeat, please go to the doctor before you try any of this stuff.

Then again, this book is about eating healthy foods. If you can die from that, then I'm gonna croak before you sue me anyway.

- Scott Davis

CONTENTS

FOREWORD

Several years ago in my book, *Live Long and Die Laughing*, I wrote a chapter entitled "My Formerly Fat Friends" featuring one of my best and most portly of buddies, Scott Davis. He appeared in that chapter because he had lost a good bit of weight. He had ulterior motives for the weight loss, as you'll see in this book, and unfortunately it didn't last. I've known Scott for almost thirty years. During those years, I've seen him go from thin in college to heavy in the '90s to "You Have Your Own Gravitational Pull" in the 21st Century. My boy was big!

He's not big anymore. This time he didn't lose weight from a pre-packaged or fad diet. Instead, he just ate for one person rather than an Army barrack, and he ate the kind of foods God intended for him to eat since he's apparently no longer training to be a Sumo wrestler.

Scott has lost more than 130 pounds. That's the size of a teenager. Can you imagine having a 14-year-old boy surgically detached from your side? Lord knows the kid is tickled to be free.

I used to visit Scott in his home outside Atlanta often. I didn't visit to see him. I went to see his mother, Mrs. Jean Davis. A few years after she passed away in 2001, Scott asked me, "Why don't you ever come visit anymore?"

"'Cause your Mama ain't there!" I said. "I went to see her, not you." It came out before I knew it.

Mrs. Davis was like a second Mama to me. She loved people and treated everyone the same. Whether you were just released from jail or you were Billy Graham, it didn't matter to her.

One of the reasons I loved Mrs. Davis is because the woman could cook! She prepared authentic, Southern feasts with fall-off-the-bone meats and vegetables cooked until they were mush. And she loved butter. Lots of butter. I'm not sure, but Paula Deen may have been her apprentice. Mrs. Davis could whip up a spread that would make your granny blush, and she did it faster than any woman I knew.

Combine her Southern cooking with lots of laughs and a warm place where you could be yourself around great company like Scott, Mrs. Jean, and

Scott's siblings, and I had a home away from home. I love stories, especially funny stories, and his family had an endless supply. Add Scott's goofy take on things, which I've always found funny, and what more could I ask for?

Over the years Scott hung out with me a lot while I toured. We discovered how much both of us love to eat. We love the flavor of food. We love the experience of trying new foods. We love the fellowship and the moment. That's where the similarities ended.

I knew when to stop. Scott would plow ahead.

When we drove from event to event, we loved looking for the out-of-the-way, hole-in-the-wall restaurants with packed parking lots. The parking lot will tell you if it's a good restaurant. If we couldn't stumble across one, we'd stop and ask the fattest person we saw. We figured we might as well consult the experts. Our motto was, "Never ask a skinny person where to eat."

Those were good times, but I grew concerned about Scott years ago. His weight and overeating spiraled out of control. He's funny—really funny. He makes me laugh. That's one reason I wanted him to be around for a while. But I knew he was digging his grave with his fork. About ten years ago, I got fed up.

"Scott, I'll give you one year to lose all that weight," I said. "If you do it, I'll give you a thousand dollars."

Did he do it? No, he got bigger, which was sad. Maybe I shouldn't have tried to bribe him, but I was willing to use drastic measures. I didn't want to lose my friend.

I live in Houston now and Scott still lives in Atlanta. We don't get to see each other like we used to. We talk on the phone and exchange emails. Shortly after he began the weight-loss approach he describes in this book, he called and told me he was going to REALLY do it this time. I rolled my eyes. After all these years and all those buffets, I thought he'd never lose the weight and would end up being a hefty challenge in the Rapture.

Then he called again. "I've lost more," he said. Then he called again. More pounds. And again. Even more pounds.

When I saw him after he had lost all the weight, I couldn't believe it. I was thrilled for my old college friend. And I was thankful he wasn't going to need reinforcements when the trumpet sounds!

You will love this book. If you are in a similar place from which Scott escaped, I pray something in these pages helps set you free. You will laugh or you might cry. Either way, you're going to have water coming out of your eyes. Consider it a start to your weight loss.

And when you reach the final page, I know for sure you will have experienced a journey of hope!

God bless you all,
Mark Lowry

Chapter 1

SQUISHING IN PUBLIC

Hotel mirrors fog up after a good, hot shower in any city, which helps when you don't want to see yourself naked. When I was big, I took long showers for two reasons. First, it took a while because I had a lot of territory to cover. Even my soap had stretch marks. Second, I didn't want to inspect the results in the mirror. Steam became my friend. A woman told me one time there's a difference between looking good and looking good naked.

Too bad that woman was my wife.

I don't even remember where I was. I just know I was late for my flight to another concert in another town. The problem with so much shower steam is it makes you hot, and I was drenched in sweat just from getting dressed. When you're 5-feet-9 and weigh more than 300 pounds, you get used to glistening in the morning even after you towel off. Sort of like pregnant women down here in the South, except we're kind enough to say they "glow."

The people mover from the airport ticketing counter to my gate wasn't working, so I had to hoof it. Had you been in the vicinity of my mad dash through the airport, you would understand why it's called *hoofing it*. I sounded like a herd of Sasquatch rumbling through Concourse B. And by then I smelled like one too.

Somewhere between ticketing and tachycardia, I had a revelation: There's a reason overweight folks struggle to find clothes that look good on them, that don't seem to show every rounded contour, that appear so form-fitting regardless of the cut of the cloth.

It's because they're usually wet.

As I reached the security station, I kicked off my slip-on shoes, whipped off my belt, unfastened my watch, and emptied my pockets. That's a lot of maneuvering for a fat boy, so it took a few moments. My heart pounded, my forehead streamed sweat, and my drenched shirt stuck to my man-boobs as I finally hustled through the metal detector.

Beeeeeeeeeeeeeeeeppppp!

I slumped my shoulders and rolled my eyes heavenward. A slight fellow who weighed maybe 155 pounds pulled me to the side. He was from the TSA, which apparently stands for Tiny Scrawny Agent. Which begs the question: What's that little dude going to do if he comes across a fat terrorist? Like he was ever going to stop Osama bin Eatin'. But I digress....

"Sir, please come with me," Mr. TSA said.

With my shoulders still slumped, I tilted my head in frustration and wheezed my way to a side section. I didn't have the energy to protest. He waved his security magic wand, and for a split second I wanted to hear "Presto!" and look down and see that he had cloned himself into my clothes. I could see myself as Mini-TSA, thin and good-looking with my spiffy—and dry—royal blue shirt.

Didn't happen. Instead, his security wand beeped.

I rolled my eyes again. Apparently I had a metal object somewhere on my very hot, very ample person. I stood with my arms outstretched, a bead of sweat puddled at the tip of my nose. I wanted to blow the sweat bead off my nose but it would've hit Mr. TSA in the face, and I was pretty sure that's a felony. I struggled to catch my breath. My arms grew heavy. My glasses fogged and I couldn't wipe them. Oh, the humanity. He waved the wand some more. I shifted my weight to the other leg as he bent down with the wand to check whether some protruding double-secret contraband had caused the weight shift.

"No, sir," I said between heaves. "That's really my calf."

I stood and panted as my heartbeat pounded in my eardrums and his wand waved and his face frowned and his beeper shrieked and people stopped in their tracks to look at this live train wreck, and I just knew the laws of physics demanded that either electrocution or spontaneous combustion occur at any second.

I held up a finger to speak but nothing came out as I sucked more air.

I wanted to beg him to let me bend over so I could catch my breath and slow the palpitations. About the time I wondered why they would even bother with an autopsy *("After a transverse dissection of the mid-thoracic cavity, subject was noted to have an unusually enlarged heart." YA THINK? I have an enlarged everything!)* Mr. TSA peered at me with the wearied look of a man about to dive into chasms and crevices never before explored. He paused and stared, as if a stark and important reminder had hit him.

He reached for the rubber gloves.

I had a doctor's office flashback and went from a hot sweat to a cold one.

As he patted me down, I couldn't help but notice him wince. When I caught my breath long enough to hear anything but my own huffing, I realized why he winced. I was squishing.

As he patted my torso, I squished every time he moved a hand to another spot on my wet shirt. And it was loud. Real loud.

Squish, squish, squish.

"OK," said Mr. TSA, a disgusted lilt in his voice. "You're clear. You can go now."

As bystanders gazed with raised eyebrows at the freak show, I realized the scene was the latest in a long line of humiliations over my ever-expanding weight.

I cracked some lame joke to move the moment along, which must've worked because he never told me what set off all the security beepers. I still don't know what caused all the fuss. I guess he figured out that, yes, those were legitimate, good ol' American rolls of fat and not a bundle of dynamite strapped around my midsection.

Mr. TSA turned toward his cohorts as I fastened everything back on to continue my rumble through the concourse. As I stepped away, Mr. TSA inadvertently caused my face to redden even more.

He looked over to a grinning co-worker and said, "I ain't never doing *that* again." The co-worker's grin turned into a giggle as I hustled away.

The thought struck me as I picked up the pace again: It's OK to poke fun at myself onstage, but life is much more pleasant when people laugh with me and not at me.

After a long, hot plane ride, I arrived at my destination and found the rental car counter. I'm notoriously cheap, so I had reserved an economy subcompact car, something just above a moped. I've gotten used to scraping my knees and elbows to wedge myself into rental Yugos over the years.

"Mr. Davis, we have reserved you a Smart Car," said the lady behind the counter.

"Great," I said. "Maybe I can just tell it where to take me and climb in the back seat for a nap."

She smiled. At least somebody humored me.

"It's in parking space A-12," she said.

Parking space A-12? That didn't sound too far away. Finally, I caught a break and didn't have far to walk. I strolled out and began looking for my Smart Car, but when I spotted it I thought it was an optical illusion.

"Does it look small because it's so far away?" I asked myself.

It wasn't an optical illusion. It was just tiny. It was one of those new-fangled, two-passenger Smart Cars that look like a cross between half a Volkswagen Bug and Darth Vader's personal spaceship. It was an egg on wheels.

"I didn't know you could drive a Tic-Tac," I said aloud. I didn't want to drive it, I wanted to eat it.

The car was cute, but I wondered how would I ever fit through the door, much less drive the thing. As I sucked in my gut, I turned to back my way inside while reaching to grab the steering wheel as a handrail. I ducked my head as far as my belly would allow and collapsed backward into the driver's seat. I'm convinced the passenger wheels came off the ground. "If I get out too fast," I asked myself, "will this car flip over?"

A jet cockpit couldn't have been any less comfortable. Even with the flexibility of a manatee, I could reach every window in the car, including the rear windshield. If I had engine trouble, I could fix it from the driver's seat. As I started down the road and found myself sucked deeper into my seat, I feared I would need the car surgically removed from my body. At least I could wear it into the O.R.

About the time I merged onto a congested interstate, with bumper-to-bumper traffic threatening my life mere feet away in either direction, I had an epiphany. While I had come to similar moments before, this time I clenched my jaw in certainty. Not that you could see my jaw line, but it was clenched. The air conditioner strained to comfort a carcass that seemed to absorb heat like a space shuttle tile, the seat groaned as it bottomed out beneath me, and my puffy face looked with new resolve into a tiny rear-view mirror of a car I wore like a suit.

"I've got to lose weight," I said to the fellow scowling back at me. "This time, I really mean it."

So I did. I lost more than 100 pounds in six months.

It was the smartest car I've ever driven.

The Reformation

Before my weight climbed to 309 pounds, when I finally put down my chubby foot and said I had to stop killing myself one bite at a time, I kept computer records. I had wanted to lose weight for years. I'd say, "I'm going to start today," and I'd be sincere but still fall off the wagon in a day or two, sometimes in just a few hours. I endured false start after false start.

At least I kept records of my past weights, recorded almost daily: 280, 284, 283, 282, 285, and on and on. When I decided once and for all to do something about my weight, I discovered that between my home computer and iPhone I had kept six years' worth of weight records.

During those six years, my weight fluctuated mostly between 260 and 280 but eventually escalated to 290. Then, at the very end, it ballooned like never before and I huffed and puffed my way to 309. I tried to be funny even at this low point. My wife, Donna, walked into the bathroom and saw me sucking in my gut as I stood on the scales.

"Honey, holding in your stomach ain't gonna make you weigh less," she said.

"I'm not holding in my stomach to weigh less," I said. "I'm trying to see the numbers."

When I had to strain sideways to read my weight, I knew I had reached the level doctors call "morbidly obese." Morbid is Latin for "You gonna be rootin' daisies before long."

I look at photographs of myself at that weight and want to cry. I was so fat that my eyes appeared swollen shut.

On November 2, 2008, at the age of 46 and roughly ten years after getting married, I started the eating plan that led to a lifestyle change that wound up changing me from the inside out. I shrank from 309 pounds to 177 pounds, a weight I had last seen in college, and achieved several objectives:

• I wanted to get healthy so I could enjoy life and live longer for my family. I was not only unhealthy but also could no longer perform many basic daily tasks without great difficulty. Or I couldn't do them at all.

• I wanted to honor God at long last by taking seriously the biblical truth that my body is a temple. If my body is a temple, then I was a megachurch, and I'd just as soon be a tiny backwoods congregation. In my fat days, the name Saddleback took on a whole new meaning.

• I wanted to do the John the Baptist thing. He said of Jesus in John 3:30: "He must increase, but I must decrease." I'm an evangelist at heart, and I don't want anything to get in the way of the Gospel, least of all that I am an undisciplined tub of goo. For Him to increase in my ministry, I had to decrease in my waistline.

I wanted to morph back into an appealing man for my wife. Yes, I was being at least partially selfish there. I like bedroom waltzes just as much as Fabio, even when I was Flabio. I wanted my wife to actually desire me again.

Those objectives fall into three important categories: physical, spiritual, and sexual. That pretty much sums up being a man. I wrote this book to chronicle a life that was roundabout in more ways than one. The fatter I grew, the further it took me from effectiveness and contentment in all of these areas.

I make no apologies that this book at times will read like an unabashed advertisement for Quick Weight Loss Centers of Atlanta (QWLCA). I owe the company my reformed life.

Quick Weight Loss Centers are independently owned clinics in various cities around the country. They are not franchised from a single corporate entity, and each may vary in approach. I have permission from QWLCA to use their name and details of my plan in this book, so I refer only to their specific approach. The Atlanta clinic has many clients monitored by phone only, meaning the QWLCA program may be used by anyone in the country.

The approach requires changing how, what, and when you eat. Doesn't any diet? The major difference is that your weight loss can be fast and substantial and is closely monitored and aided by trained staff during regular office visits or phone calls. I needed such close scrutiny not only for the accountability but also for health and safety during my monumental trek.

In Chapter Six, I detail my personal approach to healthy eating as designed by QWLCA. If you seek to lose weight and wish to use QWLCA, you will require a personalized plan as well. But the enclosed details of my plan will demonstrate how I shed 132 pounds, including more than 100 pounds in the first six months. Does it require sacrifice and incredible discipline? Yes. Does it require permanent lifestyle change to keep the weight off? You bet. Will it make a difference if once and for all you're serious and not just blowing smoke at that puffy person in the mirror? Yes.

Will it change your life? Yes, yes, and yes!

If you follow QWLCA's personal prescription, you'll not only lose weight but also re-engineer habits to enable a healthy lifestyle and permanent weight control. They taught me how to be the master rather than the slave.

For that reason alone, their approach is biblical. The health-conscious approach and the results honor God.

You may have noticed I referred to my "reformed life." Make no mistake, I'm enjoying a personal reformation. I call it Reformed Meology. I'm transformed in most physical, professional, evangelical, and even sexual aspects. I love the Lord Jesus Christ and finally decided to allow Him to have all of me. He just wanted to shrink the shell carrying me for my own good. He's the only one who could've carried me anyway. He's got the whole world in his hands, but I took up more than my fair share.

I could never say this until now: I know anyone can lose weight, even the most addictive of personalities.

Eating habits don't come any worse than the ones I had: meal after meal, drive-thru after drive-thru, snack after snack. I could've had my own cable reality show alongside all the Duggars and the dwarfs except for the fact that they couldn't fit a camera crew in the car with me.

This book will show you how you can have your own personal reformation. It doesn't have anything to do with TULIP, like Calvinism, but it has everything to do with your Two Lips.

First, you've got to speak your conviction with those Two Lips and mean it. And I'm not sporting a Gucci suit and slathering on hair gel to spout off about naming and claiming anything. The simple truth is that when it comes to what you promise yourself you finally have to get dead serious. Or you just may get dead.

Anyone can make the kind of drastic and healthy lifestyle changes I did, and that includes you—if you really want to. If you don't truly want to do it—and I mean the kind of "want to" that is a half-sister to "ticked off"—then you won't. It's that simple.

Second, if you are a believer in Christ, you have to understand that God has charged you to be the doorkeeper of those Two Lips. You have a responsibility to guard His temple.

Psalm 84:10 states that a day in God's courts is better than a thousand elsewhere. You've probably heard that phrase dozens of times in your walk with the Lord or during your time in church. But have you ever noticed the next sentence?

"I would rather be a doorkeeper in the house of my God than dwell in the tents of wickedness."

I had to make up my mind that my body, called a tent by the apostle Paul in 2 Corinthians 5:1, was nothing more than a tent of wickedness when I was a glutton enslaved to food. I'm not trying to throw guilt at you, but I want you to understand my mindset when I had my embarrassing airport escapades and later climbed off those bathroom scales and the figure 309 left me staring at the wall.

Notice I didn't stare into the mirror.

I knew I would change only if I insisted on being a doorkeeper. I would guard what I allowed in the house of my God. He indwells me. I owe Him that watch care.

The Guarantee

It dawned on me that I couldn't do it alone, however. Everyone can use help, accountability, and encouragement from a spouse or friend. Donna never had any trouble with her weight until she met me. She has never been fat, but I guess when you live with a compulsive, chronic eater for a decade, you tend to wear down and join in. Donna had put on forty pounds she wanted to shed. We often talked about trying to lose weight together, but when I saw 3-0-9 on the scales, I walked out and took over the leadership mantle that by virtue of bad habits I had abdicated years earlier.

This time, I didn't ask. Rather, I lovingly but firmly let her know we were going to lose weight. All she had to do was follow me.

Still, I realized it wasn't enough even to have Donna along for the ride. And it wasn't enough to have just another diet. I needed a lifestyle change. I needed QWLCA.

"Let's go," I told Donna. "I don't care what it costs or how long it takes. Let's go."

She didn't argue, which may have been a first, and before I knew it we were face to face with a QWLCA staff member.

"If you don't cheat," they told us, "we guarantee you that by this date you will reach your goal weight."

My goal was to reach 175 pounds. I was too big to be weighed on standard doctor's office scales, but a few feet over they had a set of cattle scales. How convenient. My embarrassment faded when I realized the cattle scales were there for a reason. I obviously wasn't the first cow they ever had to weigh. They saw my weight, crunched some numbers, and told me I'd reach my goal in about seven months, by Father's Day of 2009.

That guarantee and the visual of my reaching a weight I hadn't seen in almost 30 years—a svelte 175 pounds—was enough to solidify my resolve. I was convinced I was going to lose weight. Now I had inspiration to fuel my conviction.

It hasn't hurt that I'm able to eat a variety of foods on the QWLCA plan. It's not all one focus, like a diet with no carbs or all rice or all protein. It's balanced. I eat fruits, vegetables, meats, dairy, and grains. I have limitations and foods to avoid, but my meals are varied enough that I don't worry about cravings or monotony driving me back to Fatdom.

The QWLCA team guaranteed a weight loss of three to five pounds a week. On my way to losing my first 100 pounds, I averaged losing about four pounds per week. The bigger you are, the quicker it comes off at first. Maybe it's because it's mostly excess water. I lost 10 pounds the first week, and I could feel a little slack in my pants, shirts, and belt. Once I explain my personality a little more in later chapters, you'll understand why such instant gratification motivated me to keep going.

People ask me how much I exercised to lose so much weight. Here's the exciting part for overweight folks....

I lost 132 pounds *without exercising*. In losing my first 30 pounds, I couldn't bend over, much less exercise. I'm exercising some now, but all I did to lose weight was eat right.

I can't stress enough that I didn't starve myself either. I didn't eat too little, and I didn't lose weight too fast. This was because I ate vegetables, fruit, and protein every day. I even drank coffee. I ate like one person *should* eat. I used to eat enough food for three people. Or a small village on some days.

You know how people who have lost weight say they feel better and more alive? Well, I discovered the reason for the cliché. It's true.

I do feel better. I go to bed earlier and wake earlier. Discipline in one area has led to discipline in other areas. I'm more consistent in my quiet time with the Lord. I have more energy. I actually *want* to take the trash to the road now.

The QWLCA plan lived up to its name, and my quick weight loss stoked my fire to stick with it.

Some people want to know why my goal weight was 175 pounds. Mark Hall from Casting Crowns is a friend who serves as student pastor at my church and also travels with me to help conduct student conferences at Christian schools. He saw me before I reached my goal weight and said, "Why do you want to lose more? You look fine the way you are."

Maybe. I've learned that you can cover up a lot with clothes, but some places need all the help they can get. The reason for the goal weight of 175 is more symbolic than anything else. It comes with a token, a prop, for motivation.

In my homesick freshman year at Liberty Baptist College (now Liberty University), I tried out for a traveling group called SMITE. The horrible name meant Student Missionary Intern Training for Evangelism. I know, it's weird: *"Come hear all about the grace of God with the SMITE singers."*

I wondered if we would go around hitting people: "I smite thee in the name of the Lord!" They've since changed it to Light Ministries, which makes more sense. It's a missions team, and we traveled to thirteen countries and ministered with Dr. Jerry Falwell, the founder of Liberty, and SMITE director Roscoe Brewer.

During the time I traveled with SMITE, we stopped in Hong Kong. I discovered I could get a quality suit tailored cheaply there, and I bought a custom-made suit in Hong Kong when I weighed 175 pounds.

Before my QWLCA transformation, I found that suit in my closet. I stumbled across it just after my defining moment when I said, "I've got to do something once and for all about my weight." I stopped and stared at the coat, my mind flashing back to Hong Kong and the sweet little guy who took my measurements.

I said to myself, "I'm going to get into this again."

Less than a year later, I put on the jacket while weighing 177 pounds, two pounds shy of my weight on the day I had the coat tailored in Hong Kong. The coat has moth holes and it's out of style, but it fits me. I admit it's still a little snug.

But it won't be for long.

Chapter 2

GOLDEN NUGGETS

Mark Lowry and I missed a good chance to be twins. Not that he's ever been rotund, but our life paths are remarkably similar. I think that's why we became such good buddies despite the fact I'm so much funnier and better looking than he is. Sometimes I have to work to draw him out of his shell.

We both make our livings as Christian humorists and singers. We both are Southern boys. We both attended Liberty. We both suffer from common maladies. Mark is open about his battle with ADD, and I've always had an ADD problem too. I *add* a lot of helpings to my plate and I *add* a lot of items to my buggy and I *add* a lot of toppings on my dessert.

Mark is best known for his work with the Gaither Vocal Band, but we've passed a lot of mile markers together. I appeared in several of his videos, wrote for him, and hung out with him on some of his tours.

When I visit our old college town of Lynchburg, Virginia, I often stay with Mark's parents. His father, Charles, is an attorney who was on retainer for Dr. Jerry Falwell. According to Mark, that was enough to keep his dad with a full-time job. Mark's mother, Bev, taught psychology at Liberty. They have an apartment in their basement, which allows me to stay at least one night on the road for free. I'm cheap, so I'm fond of the arrangement. Plus, I get to fellowship with old friends and escape another sterile and lonely hotel room. One year, I wound up wishing I'd splurged on the hotel room.

The Lowrys have a beautiful home. In their basement apartment is a nice bathroom, a veritable sanctuary for a man who values the peace of a daily constitutional. In that nice bathroom is a fine commode. And on that fine commode during my visit was a bit of an indulgence for a man who values the peace of a daily constitutional. It had a comfortable, smooth, expensive-looking wooden seat.

I don't know if it was mahogany, walnut, hickory, oak, pine, or glossed-over particleboard, but it sure felt good. Especially for such a wide expanse.

I have to preface this story by saying the wooden seat was already cracked a little before I sat on it. I just want you to know that.

Somewhere within the tranquility of the moment—probably about Page 2-B of *The Lynchburg News and Advance*—something popped beneath me. The snapping sound reached my brain a split second before the searing pain did. It was something akin to a hornet sting in a very bad place.

I yelped like a coonhound.

When that seat snapped underneath my weight, just enough flesh wedged into the crack of the seat that it left an indelible mark way too close to the crack of *my* seat. It's not easy to dance when your pants are around your ankles. I managed to keep my balance as I flailed and rubbed.

I shined my bottom toward the mirror to check whether I had a gaping wound. Gaping, yes. Wound, no. I had only a small red mark surrounding a rising white welt.

I found myself in a bit of a bind. Upstairs, my hosts surely heard the commotion and wondered whether they needed to dial 911 to stop the burglary in progress downstairs. What could I do—act like it didn't happen? I couldn't exactly play it off. Broken hardware was involved, and duct tape would've been too obvious.

So I did what any good comedian would do. I grabbed the broken half of the seat and waddled upstairs.

"Mr. Lowry!" I yelled as I held up the seat. "Ummm. Your seat broke."

He looked up, shook his head, and laughed. Thank God for the Lowry humor gene. Such is life for a fat man. You live. You learn. You break things. And you laugh a lot, especially when it's such an effective front.

Bless his heart, Mark Lowry bore the burden of my weight more than once. One year, my mother and I visited him at his home when he lived in Nashville. The guest room featured two antique twin beds. I slept in one bed and mom slept in the other. The beds were gifts to Mark from a well-known Christian singer. They were old...like, Bunker Hill old. They popped and creaked when you rolled over. It was a natural alarm clock when somebody shifted in the other bed.

My bed groaned under my girth, begging for relief that finally came sometime in the middle of the night. As I flopped over on my side, the foot of the bed collapsed to the floor. The concussion rattled the walls. My mom muttered something—I was too incoherent to make it out—but my size paled in comparison to my laziness. I didn't try to fix it. Too groggy to lose sleep over it, I inclined myself with my head up and my feet near the floor for the rest of the night.

The next morning I thought, "Great. I broke Mark's bed, and not just any bed but a gift from a famous singer. I assumed Mark heard the loud crash and called his parents to whisper, 'Tubby did it again.'"

Another time, I broke my own guest bed at home. I grew so big and snored so loudly that I had to sleep in our guest bedroom to enable Donna to get some rest. Plus, I stayed hot and sweaty all night and Donna suffered from hot flashes at the time. She felt she was the source of global warming and just knew Al Gore would track her down. My heat combined with her heat was too much. She let me know she wasn't sleeping in the Easy-Bake Oven another night.

One night I turned over in the guest bed and a whole side of the bed fell off of the frame and thudded to the floor. Once again, I didn't budge. I just wallowed around and slept uphill so I wouldn't fall out.

I laughed off such incidents, but the reality is they happened. And they happened for one reason. I was fat.

People who saw me gorge myself always asked me, "Why do you eat like that?" I have an acquaintance named Marty McCall who sang with the group First Call, which provided backup for Sandi Patty. Marty joined Mark Lowry and me at a Gospel Music Association meeting many years ago. We weaved through the booths on the convention floor, and as they heard my wheezing for breath the subject soon turned to my obvious weight problem.

Once Marty realized I was comfortable with the topic, he opened up: "Why are you so big? There has to be a reason. What motivates you to *stay* big? Why don't you lose weight? There has to be some mental or psychological reason for you to be this way." He asked these questions in the flow of the conversation and wasn't being rude or too forward. I wracked my brain but couldn't come up with an answer right then.

For years, I thought about those questions. Why was I so fat, so enamored with food, so utterly lost about what to do about it? Had I been abused as a child? Did somebody shove Twinkies down my throat in nursery school, or what? There was nothing I could pinpoint. I've just always loved food.

I've had people tell me you're supposed to eat until you're full. It was their subtle way of encouraging me to moderate. I always replied with my motto: "Well, you've got to plow past full. If it tastes good, you push through that full barrier and keep going."

I eat for the pleasure of it. A lot of people suffer addictions—drugs, alcohol, pornography, sex, the Internet. Food makes me feel good. It's my drug of choice. I enjoy the taste of it. I enjoy feeling full. I enjoy having something in my mouth. I'm sure Freud wrote a very boring volume about that somewhere. Admittedly, I got to the point where I felt miserable and wanted to wear only stretchy pants.

We'd head out to a restaurant, and I'd think, "I'm putting on my sweatpants because this one is all-you-can-eat."

I'm sure lineage played a part in my obesity, but not as you may think (as I will show you in a few chapters). I've heard big people use the line, "I feel like there's a thin person on the inside trying to get out."

Not me. I was just the opposite. My umbilical cord was fat. Even when I was trim as a child and physically fit in college, I felt like I had a fat person on the inside trying to get out. Yet I refuse to use lineage as a scapegoat. As I will explain, my primary problem of horrific eating habits started in college and blossomed into full-blown addiction as an adult.

First Corinthians 19:20 says, "Do you not know that your body is the temple of the Holy Spirit, who is in you, whom you have from God, and you are not your own? For you were bought at a price; therefore, glorify God in your body and in your spirit, which are God's."

The same Paul who calls my body a tent in 2 Corinthians 5:1 also calls it a temple in 1 Corinthians 3:16. One description deals with the frailty and impermanence of the human condition, and the other proclaims the majestic truth that the Holy Spirit permanently makes our hearts His home—His temple.

It's easy to skim past a key phrase in that last sentence: "Therefore, glorify God in your body." I often glorified God in my words. I told people about Jesus. I shared my faith. I just didn't share my dessert. If you reached over toward my plate, you might've drawn back a nub. I certainly didn't glorify God in my body, though I came awfully close to being named the Eighth Wonder of the World.

I finally made a commitment to QWLCA because I had to do something. My life was at stake. And Lord knows I'd tried just about everything else.

Diet Roulette

The unspoken prayer request of all fat people is that they've just started a new diet. It's a part of life.

I lost count of how many diets I tried over the years. If somebody was pitching the latest craze, I was buying. One year, I was on five diets at once just to get enough to eat. I loved the liquid diet because I figured out how to do a roast beef smoothie...with a biscuit-and-gravy chaser.

I've told that joke before at some conservative churches and they laughed but stared at me, grinning with eyes widened, because they couldn't believe I said the word "chaser" in church. That's barroom lingo.

Lutheran churches don't care. They understand.

I became desperate for a diet that would work. Technically, I was desperate for a diet that would work while still permitting my horrible eating habits. I wanted somebody to invent a weight loss pill called "Sleep-Away."

When I'm home from the road, I'm usually tired. At home, I like to be sedentary because I make a living on the move. I often park in my recliner in front of the TV, sometimes well into the night.

I love watching QVC and the Home Shopping Network. Donna is different. She likes department stores and malls. She'll shop for hours in what must be some feminine therapeutic ritual I'll never understand. I accused her of shopping too much the other day.

"Who do you think I am, Bill Cosby? Have you checked the mailbox for the royalties lately?"

I could hear her huff behind me.

"You're addicted to shopping too," she said. "You're just too lazy to get off the couch and go to the store."

Point taken. I am lazy, which is a huge part of my huge problem. I sat watching TV a few nights ago and the remote control lay on the floor just out of arm's reach.

"This show is boring," I said to no one in particular. Then I looked at the out-of-reach remote, paused for a moment, and said, "Well, I'll give it a chance."

You can see why the diets didn't work.

I tried Deal-a-Meal after watching Richard Simmons sob his way through an infomercial. I made fun of the guy, of course. He acted so sweet with his big, bouffant hairdo and high, silky shorts. But then halfway through the program I pulled out the Visa and dialed the 1-800 number. Six to eight weeks later I received a deck of cards in the mail.

Now understand, I grew up in a strict, fundamental, 1611 King James Version-only independent Baptist church. We didn't go to movies. We didn't dance. And we definitely didn't play cards. But I learned how to play cards with that Deal-a-Meal deck because it had pictures of food on it.

Donna would pull a card and show it to me.

Broccoli.

Broccoli? I grunted and shook my head.

"Hit me."

Cauliflower?

"Hit me again. I'm going for the cheesecake."

The deck allotted a certain number of cards for each meal. You don't eat the cards, but they tell you what to eat. I ran out of cards by 9 a.m.

I looked over at Donna and said, "Get me another deck."

I tried the Hollywood Grapefruit Diet. It helps if you like grapefruit. Plus, I worried I'd wind up like all the emaciated starlets in Hollywood who need to eat a sandwich. I think I'd rather be fat than be able to count my bones and veins and trip over my swollen lips. Of course, no one would be able to detect my misery since my face would be Botoxed into a permanent smile like the Joker from Batman.

> I realized the only diet worth trying is one I could maintain the rest of my life.

I downloaded a diet off the Internet in which I ate only cabbage soup for three days. The instructions didn't say anything about flatulence. I was self-propelled for days. Besides, try living off cabbage soup two or three times a day. Cabbage soup today. Cabbage soup tomorrow. Here a cabbage, there a cabbage, everywhere a cabbage cabbage. Did I really think that would work? It tasted halfway decent only with a couple of sleeves of soda crackers or a slab of cornbread, which defeated the purpose.

I realized the only diet worth trying is one I could maintain the rest of my life. I didn't need another Band-Aid covering the scratch where I itched for a few impassioned days. I needed a heart transplant. The change had to stick.

Speaking of sticking…

I once tried a Chocolate-and-Milk diet. I took Ex-Lax and washed it down with Milk of Magnesia. I sat on the toilet for a week. I sat there so long my butt went to sleep. It's a moment you'll never forget when your tail tingles. I was stuck to the commode and had to rock back and forth to get the blood flowing to my legs so I could stand.

I even tried the Atkins Diet. I loved it for a while because it allows a lot of foods I like to eat. But it's all meat and little or no bread, pastas, and "white foods." That got old, and then came the nasty media controversy over whether it was a healthy alternative.

One of the reasons I like the QWLCA plan is it permits real food and is balanced among the major food groups. Still, when people approach me and ask me about this plan, I tell them I realized the only effective diet would have to start in my mind. It had to be a mental thing, because every diet out there will work if you really want it to work.

That includes Weight Watchers, which rates foods on a points system and allocates the dieter so many points a day and so many flex points a week. I found out those flex points don't roll over like cell phone minutes. You can't save up those suckers for later. You have to use them.

After one of my concerts, my music partner, Billy Lord, and road manager, Eric Jackson, joined me at a restaurant. I don't know if many men have a tendency to spill food on themselves when they eat, but I do. As I burrowed into my meal, it dawned on me that I was on Weight Watchers. And I was binging again.

Billy swallowed a bite and sat up in his seat, craning to look over the table. He motioned with a finger.

"You've got a little something on your shirt," he said.

I looked down and frowned.

"I've got more points on my shirt than I'm supposed to have for the whole week," I said. "So *there's* the third course."

I have nothing personal against Weight Watchers. Great company. But Weight Watchers wasn't ideal for me because they guaranteed I'd lose a pound a week. My attention span is short. I need instant gratification. I like TiVo because I can watch my show right now. I love the microwave. I love the iPhone. I want to see results yesterday. A mere pound a week didn't cut it. I needed bigger results and a suddenly smaller waistline to see something worth the pursuit.

I couldn't find a plan that motivated me enough to stick with it until I found QWLCA. Theirs was the only approach that broke a nasty cycle miring my every previous attempt. That cycle became my seven deadly sins of weight control. In this book, I share my experiences, mistakes, and lessons at each of those seven stages to offer folks in similar situations a way of escape.

Golden Nuggets

I love chicken nuggets, especially crispy ones. 'Course, I would gnaw on them even if they were sopping wet with grease. I thought of chicken nuggets when I remembered the seven steps I used to lose weight. Don't get your hopes up. I haven't invented a cure-all chicken nugget diet, but there was a time when I'd been willing to try that one too.

While I've proven I can master a diet and lose major weight, that's not what I'm good at. I'm good at eating—really good. And not just eating anything but eating everything, especially stuff that tastes terrific and pumps you full of artery glue.

In the spirit of the awful habits from which I escaped, I propose seven steps certain to work miracles for your waistline—if you want to keep expanding. I call them *Golden Nuggets: Seven Sure-Fried Ways to Stay Fat or Get Even Fatter*. They're in jest, of course, but you'll get the idea as we go along. Just do the opposite of what I did for most of my adult life while pursuing these steps that have a profound (and round) effect on your waistline, and you'll probably lose a lot of weight and live a long time.

Golden Nuggets: Seven Sure-Fried Ways to Stay Fat or Get Even Fatter

Swallow the Truth
Enjoy the Freedom Fries
Welcome to Waffle House
Supersize It—with a Large Diet Coke, Please
Fly Solo: Where Even the Airplane Food Tastes Good
Dessert Your Will
Place Your Order Anywhere But at the Lord's Table

I used to think a one-size-fits-all formula for weight loss didn't exist and if I had one Bill Gates would be my butler. And this would be the last diet book ever published.

But the truth is this *could* be the last diet book ever published. If everyone ate as healthy as the QWLCA plan ascribes, all the other diet plans would go out of business. Meaningful and lasting weight control is about eating healthy.

If you struggle with weight control or overeating like I did, I encourage you to unlearn these seven steps. You'll have to walk with me through the next seven chapters to examine how each of these changed my life and how, with God's help, I regained control at each vicious stage. Believe me, it was a God-sized task.

It all began with that first step: *Swallow the Truth.* That's where the Lord met with me in the most personal of ways, tapped me on my fleshy shoulder, and curled His finger at me to put down the burrito and come to Him.

Chapter 3

BOTH CHEEKS FULL
"Swallow the Truth"

I've studied the Bible enough to know the temple in Jerusalem featured large courts as gathering places for different groups of people. King Solomon's Temple, destroyed by the Babylonians around 586 B.C., had two major courts, the Great Court and the Inner Court. Jesus visited Herod's Temple, destroyed by the Romans in 70 A.D. It featured several courts, including the Court of the Gentiles, the Court of the Women, the Court of the Priests, and the Court of the Israelites.

If you'd seen me a few years ago, you'd have known my temple had a food court.

The first of my seven slim-proof Golden Nuggets will do wonders to keep any personal temple in dire need of remodeling.

Swallow the Truth.

For years, I swallowed the truth and everything else I could get my hands on. I refused to admit I had a problem, especially in one intensely personal way I will detail later in this chapter.

I told myself my eating habits were fine. All I would admit to was, yes, I had a spaghetti stain on my shirt. I rationalized in ways that now seem laughable: If God didn't put all those burgers, fries, and desserts on Earth to enjoy, then why did He make them so finger-lickin' good? I had different ideas on displaying the *full* Gospel. As large as I was, it didn't get any more full. I saw no sense in talking about the 500-pound elephant in the room, especially since I was the elephant.

I knew the truth because I knew God's Word. But I wouldn't admit the truth because I loved my addiction more than I loved doing the right thing. It led to one place.

It led to a personal hell.

The War

Have you ever noticed the root word of diet is *die?*

I'm not sure if that has a physical or spiritual connotation, or both. I know it feels like you're going to die when you're big and starving yourself. I know sometimes you think you're dying for a bite to eat. But I think the spiritual implication is more appropriate. To diet is to die to self in a real way, a way that can make a fat person camp out in Romans 6 and 7.

I can't tell you how many times I planned to die to self when it came to food. I would say, "OK, this is the day. I'm gonna lose the weight starting right now." Every single time—thousands of them—I had only honest, good intentions of following through.

I would start out great, going most of the day without a morsel or perhaps eating certain foods to obey the diet du jour. But then it happened. For some reason I've yet to comprehend, I stumbled. I ate something not on my list and invariably felt I blew it.

"Well, I've messed up, so I might as well eat whatever I want today," I said. "I can start the diet fresh tomorrow."

Ah, the twisted logic of a fat man staring at a cabinet full of Little Debbies.

Here's the wicked irony: Because I knew I would start over the next day, I awarded myself permission not just to eat but to go crazy for the rest of the day. It's not an exaggeration to say on some days I scarfed down nearly every edible item in sight. I felt half bulimic. I had the binging part down.

My work schedule didn't help. I faced constant battles at home and on the road.

I don't have what most folks would consider a real job, but I am self-employed. I set my own schedule, a dangerous freedom when you have a size 50-plus waist. While at home, I constantly run errands to maintain my ministry and home. I make runs to the post office, bank, Wal-Mart, and Office Depot (I can at least fantasize about being neat and organized, can't I?).

For most people this would be a routine afternoon, but for me it was the battleground of my two warring halves: Supersize Scotty and Skinny Scotty.

Supersize Scotty usually won, turning the afternoon jaunt into a perverted feast. Between each errand during my fat years, I wheeled into the drive-thru of the closest fast-food restaurant. *Between each errand.*

At McDonald's I ordered the $1 double cheeseburger. Supersize Scotty chirped into action.

"Hey, it's only a dollar, so it won't matter much."

Skinny Scotty wagged his finger: "Uh, price has nothing to do with calorie count, big boy."

Many times, since the double cheeseburger cost little, I inhaled two of them. On my worst days, I threw in a Big Mac on top of the double cheeseburgers, and Supersize Scotty grinned with both cheeks full.

Chowing and driving, I pulled into the post office, tossed the sack of empty wrappers into the trash, checked my mail, and took off again. After the McDonald's meal, I still felt hungry, or at least thought I did, and Krystal beckoned. Again, in my addicted and illogical thinking, I talked myself into stopping. Supersize Scotty sat on my left shoulder and whispered, "The burgers are so little that they're not even burgers. They're bites. No harm."

Skinny Scotty sat on my right shoulder and dreamed of doing pushups again one day. "Don't do it!" he screamed. "Don't listen to Chunkalicious over there!"

Chunkalicious always won. My routine included four little Krystals and two Chili Pups. I washed them down with my second Diet Coke. It was a diet drink, after all. Skinny Scotty giggled at the fallacy.

I strolled through Office Depot and dreamt of becoming a disciplined and compartmentalized wonder, then took off to the next stop and ignored a stark truth. I had compartmentalized my eating. I had concocted a kingdom fortified with almost impenetrable lies.

To get back home I had to drive past one last temptation. Supersize Scotty loved burritos. He also loved seafood. He had the best of both worlds at the final outpost on my way home: a Taco Bell/Long John Silver's combo restaurant. Skinny Scotty told me he never understood how anyone could mix fish and Mexican food, but by then he sounded like Charlie Brown's teacher. *Wahh Wahh Wonk, Wonk Wahh Wahh.*

Is there such thing as a bad meal?

By the time I made it home, almost full and forever unfulfilled, I lumbered from the car thick with the smell and chemical haze of fast food, a man drained by the hell of battle. I'd walk in the front door after running a few errands, and Donna would say, "Why were you gone for four hours?"

I felt like Paul in Romans 7. I had the desire to do right but felt completely defeated to be able to carry it out. I didn't do the good I wanted to do but rather the evil I loathed.

And loved.

In the end, neither Supersize Scotty nor Skinny Scotty was happy. They plopped on either shoulder, arms folded and brows furrowed, wondering when I'd ever truly listen. And deep down, it was all I could do to keep from screaming "O wretched man that I am! Who will deliver me from this body of death?" (Romans 7:24).

Double Jeopardy

The Bible says God made some vessels for wrath and some vessels for mercy. (Romans 9:22-23) I praise the Lord for His grace because on some days I felt cursed. Being fat and cheap is a double-whammy. Those two weaknesses are a lethal mixture. I needed a Surgeon General's warning sticker on my forehead:

IMITATING THIS FREAK IS DANGEROUS TO YOUR HEALTH!

Donna tells me I'm cheap and tacky. I love to shop at Wal-Mart. She likes fancy stores like Dillard's and Macy's. Usually, in concert everything I wear has a tag on the back that reads "Faded Glory." Wal-Mart people know exactly what I'm talking about. What Donna calls cheap I call frugal. I like being a good steward, but for some reason she grew incensed when I bought her a bag of generic cheese puffs. That's the white bag with the black letters that read, "CHEESE PUFFS" in block letters. Underneath in small print it says, "Or may be used as packing material." She didn't appreciate that at all.

I guess sometimes I carry my penny-pinching a bit far. If Suave would make a car I'd drive it.

I'm also a man of convenience, meaning I often fulfill Donna's labels of cheap and tacky. It seems like every time I want something she says, "You're going to have to build a whole 'nother room for that," because she doesn't want it in the house.

For instance, I want the fake fish that hangs on the wall and it turns its head to sing to you. She won't let me buy it. One Christmas season, Wal-Mart had a fake deer head at the front of the store. It sang Jingle Bells as you walked in.

"Now that'd look good in the foyer," I said.

She shook her head and never slowed down as she spoke over her shoulder. "You'll get it when Jingle Bells freezes over."

I want one of those double recliners. It's a giant L-shaped sofa with recliners on either end. We have a nice house, and I know the double recliners seem to fit perfectly in the floor plan for a trailer, but for some reason she won't let me have stuff like that. She likes the finer things. I want that double recliner so I can lower the middle console and put my Big Gulp in the cupholder, plug up my cell phone, and situate my remote control at a perfect angle. I want one with a seat warmer and a vibrating back massager. If it had a toilet built into it, I might not ever get up. I could hang my fish right above it and have a sing-along. Donna didn't say I'd need a whole 'nother room for that. She said I'd need a whole 'nother house. I got the hint.

I like bargains. I like sales. I like shopping at Goodwill. So what if the shirt came off a dead guy? It's two dollars.

Problem is, the cheap mindset is a killer for an obese person. Something cheap or easy typically means it's low quality or unhealthy. Notice how I called myself a man of convenience earlier. Translation: I'm bone-lazy.

All of this rendered my little living room nest Ground Zero for my bad habits.

I went through stretches in which I lived like a vampire. I stayed up to the wee hours, gorged myself, and slept late the next day. Sometimes I went all day on a well-meaning diet but still unleashed the hungry hounds when the sun went down. Television wasn't nearly as appealing without something to munch on. I made my spiral into the depths of bad habits easier when I propped up my feet.

Once again, I started out with good intentions. At first I ate only half a banana. I grabbed the 45-calorie diet bread and thought, "This can't be bad." But it always worsened.

"OK, if my bread is only 45 calories, then a little peanut butter won't hurt," I thought. "Oooh, you know what? Maybe I'll mix a little honey on top of that."

Then I added the half-banana, the healthy ingredient that got the dough-ball rolling in the first place. I had a way of making even naturally healthy foods unhealthy. Then I drank a half-glass of skim milk to just make sure I stayed on the diet.

It was as if the snack got my stomach juices flowing.

I fixed another half-sandwich like the previous one and thought, "It can't be that bad. It's only 45 calories for this and 40 calories for that. It's a banana and peanuts. It's real, natural food."

Before long, I lost all restraint. I started with a teaspoon of peanut butter, and then I switched to a tablespoon. Then I went to the ice cream scoop and jammed it into the Jif jar. I grabbed the little honey container shaped like a bear and squeezed him until he had pain on his face. I whipped the peanut butter and honey into a wonderful goo and spread it all over the bread. The goo was thicker than the bread. I washed it down with another glass of milk (skim milk, mind you). Then I made another goo sandwich and sucked down another glass of milk.

Finally, I finished off the other half of the banana. I knew it was good for me and would go bad if I didn't eat it. I just couldn't let it spoil.

My biggest weakness was cereal. I even went with plain shredded wheat without the icing for the health factor. Shredded wheat has to be better for you than Count Chocula, right?

Not with me. I literally piled 10 packs of artificial sweetener on top. My shredded wheat looked like snow-capped mountains. I'd be on some diet that called for shredded wheat with a half-cup of skim milk for breakfast, and yet I'd eat it at midnight and pour in enough milk to float a canoe. When the cereal ran out before the milk, I poured in more cereal so I wouldn't waste the milk. And when the milk ran low and the second bowl of cereal became too dry, I couldn't waste the cereal so I poured in more milk. The unrelenting cycle of rationalization left me wiping milk off my chin after the fifth bowl.

I ate a whole sleeve of Ritz Crackers and peanut butter. I grubbed to the back of a nearly empty pantry and found a can of chili with beans, the kind with the nasty orange gel on top when you open the can. I warmed it just enough to melt the gel.

Then I switched to Saltine Crackers and tuna because I was down to the last can standing. Same formula: Start with a few crackers and some tuna. Then eat a few more, always a few more. Then pour a few cans of tuna into a bowl, mix it with a vat of real, whole, gooey mayonnaise, and plow in with more crackers. Then throw in some relish to spice up my snack, which looked more like my third meal in an hour.

I did this over and over and over until I went to bed or fell asleep face-first in my cereal. If I was awake, I had to put something in my mouth or plan for it.

During Thanksgiving and Christmas holidays, I went ballistic. I love homemade sweet potato pies without much spice. My mother would make one and I'd get a little sliver, thinking it wouldn't hurt anything. The addiction engine roared to life.

"Man, that went down good," I thought. "I only had a little sliver. And it's a sweet potato, which is natural. It has to be good for you. It came out of the ground."

Yes, and so does opium.

I sliced another sliver only to cut it crooked and think, "Oh, I've got to straighten that out. I can't leave the pie looking like that."

I cut wider to straighten the edge. Supersize Scotty was alive and suffering from OCD.

Sometimes Donna bought her favorite dessert: yellow cake with butter cream icing. The grocery store bakery encases cakes in a clear plastic container. The lid pops and crackles when you pry it open, which isn't good for a thick-fingered sneak. When Donna fell asleep, I tried to be quiet so she couldn't hear me getting into the cake. I learned to adapt. I used a blanket to cover the cake container and muffle the noise while I tugged and pried.

"All right, if I can just take a quarter-inch slice," I thought, "that's not much."

But when a cake is fifteen inches wide, a quarter-inch slice is a slab. I scraped the leftover icing and crumbs from around the rim and licked my finger.

Donna caught me a couple of times. She knew I was supposed to watch my weight, so I always snuck something and tried to hide the evidence. This is pitiful to admit: I often dug through the trash to put the fresh snack wrapper underneath all the other trash so she wouldn't see it. She still found the wrapper a few times and nailed me.

"I know you had three candy bars," she said the next day.

I've told that story in my comedy routine and discovered other people have used the same sneaky method to cloak their binging from spouses. I always had a joke ready because the mood was the only thing I could manage to lighten.

"Honey, we need clear plates," I responded when she caught me. "When

I'm done eating I can lick my plate and still see the TV. I won't miss a thing on either one."

She laughed. I laughed. And Supersize Scotty cackled again, smacking and licking his thumb, both cheeks full.

Revelation

The first stage in any change is admitting change is needed. The human mind has an incredible capacity to assent to something without taking it personally or buying into it. For me, nothing changed until my admission became intensely personal.

I had to admit I was an addict.

I had to admit I couldn't control myself without help.

Worst of all, I had to admit I was sinning against a holy God. I was out of God's will.

The Apostle James says each person is tempted when he is lured and enticed by his own desire. (James 1:14) It comes from within. It comes from me. I'm to blame.

When it dawned on me that I sinned against God by binging, overeating at every meal, and eating unhealthy foods habitually, only then did I begin to think I could forge monumental change.

The last thing I want to do is sound preachy in this book. Lord knows, just because I had to punch a few new holes in my belt doesn't give me more room to judge. I grew up in an independent Baptist church, and it wasn't unusual to see an obese preacher or evangelist. When you're threatening the 500-pound barrier, you really have no business pounding the pulpit and throwing spit about someone drinking, smoking, doing drugs, or listening to rock music. It's hard to listen to a holy roller when you can't get past his unholy rolls.

That also convicted me. I travel all over the country to perform and make people laugh, but another crucial element of my shows is a presentation of the Gospel of Jesus Christ. I am an evangelist. My ministry is sharing Christ, and my tools are comedy and song.

I didn't know the definition of weight until I realized I couldn't let my light shine before others because my big body kept getting in the way. I was a walking eclipse. Now *that* was heavy.

Imagine how awkward I felt, especially considering how I viewed the fat preachers of my youth, as I stood onstage for 100-plus shows per year. Night after night I told thousands of people about the narrow way. I felt guilty even as I shared the truth, knowing if we traveled the narrow road together I needed a WIDE LOAD banner across my front and my own escort car with a flashing yellow light.

One of my life's theme verses is Acts 20:24: "But none of these things move me; nor do I count my life dear to myself, so that I may finish my race with joy, and the ministry which I received from the Lord Jesus, to testify to the gospel of the grace of God."

> I felt guilty even as I shared the truth, knowing if we traveled the narrow road together I needed a WIDE LOAD banner across my front and my own escort car with a flashing yellow light.

Just before that verse, Paul explains that everywhere he had gone God made it clear to him through the Holy Spirit that "chains and tribulations" awaited him. He knew he was headed to some sort of confinement for his faith.

When I read "but none of these things move me," I thought, "Well, how can that be? How could Paul know he was bound for prison and not haul tail the other way?"

It's because he wasn't his own. He owed his life to someone else. I would make that point in concert but still couldn't help but think…

Same with me when it comes to food. I'm not my own. I'm enslaved.

The sticking point with a lot of people when it comes to salvation is they first must realize they're lost. They have to get lost so they can get saved. They're good people who don't see the need for a Savior.

I believe the Bible is true. I'm like the old preacher I heard one time. He said, "I believe from Genesis all the way to the maps." At one point, Jesus says, "I am the way, the truth, and the life. No one comes to the Father except through me." (John 14:6) That really doesn't have to be explained. It's pretty blunt. He's the answer. Sometimes people believe the existence of Jesus and even believe he's the Son of God. Yet they don't believe they need Him because they don't believe they're bad enough to need Him. And then again I looked at my gut and thought….

Same with me when it comes to food.

A couple of years ago, Fox News reported survey results in which eighty-five percent of Americans believed they would go to heaven when they die. But fifty percent of those same people said Jesus wasn't the only way to heaven and that someone could reach heaven by practicing Buddhism, Hinduism, Islam or by just being good.

That's not what Jesus says. He claims exclusivity.

I've conducted or taken part in a lot of evangelistic events, and I've found that most people believe the Bible is true—whether they're churched or unchurched. So if you believe the Bible is true, then you believe what Jesus said about Himself. He's the only way to heaven. He's the only way to get where you really want to go.

Same with me when it comes to food.

The Bible goes on to say, "For with the heart one believes unto right-eousness, and with the mouth confession is made unto salvation" (Romans 10:10) and "whoever calls upon the name of the Lord shall be saved" (Romans 10:13).

It's not enough to know the facts. It has to be transferred to our hearts. It's a heart decision.

Same with me when it comes to food.

Once we realize Jesus is the only way to heaven, the only wise response is to say, "Jesus, I'm a sinner. Please forgive me of my sins and come into my life and take over. I'm doing a one-eighty with my life and turning to you. I surrender. Be the Lord of my life."

For some reason, a stigma has been attached to the term "born again." It simply means we allow Jesus to be the boss who sets us on a new path.

Same with me when it comes to food.

The aforementioned Acts 20:24 says, "so that I may finish my race with joy," comparing the Christian life with a race headed toward the finish line of heaven. I don't complain about God's Word because it is truth. But it talks an awful lot about running. And I don't like running, even though I run every morning at 7 a.m.

I run from the bed to the bathroom and then back to the bed.

When we accept Christ, the Holy Spirit moves into our hearts. He takes up residence inside us and never goes away. That's why Paul was unmoved by the threat of imprisonment for his faith in Christ. He had surrendered his life to the Holy Spirit's control. When we have the Holy Spirit in our lives, such threats and fears are muted by the sweet peace of a Savior who bears our burdens.

Most people don't get up in the morning and say, "I'm going to be a heathen today." Instead, most people when they become a Christian say, "God, I'm going to give everything to you. All these challenges are yours. Except for this one little area. I've got to hang onto it. This is too good. I can't part with this."

Same with me when it comes to food.

We have to give it *all* to God whether it's our thought life, where we go, what we do, what we listen to and watch, what we look at on the computer, and, in many cases, what we eat. When I talked with God about the stuff I faced, first on the list was the face I stuffed.

I had to allow God through His Holy Spirit to take control of the one area in which I had dug huge bunkers and erected massive fortifications—the seemingly pedestrian, practical function of what I fed myself each day. I was blinded by my sin even though overeating or eating poorly isn't a sin I could hide very well. A quick glance in the mirror revealed just how far short of the glory of God I had fallen, which was the reason I hated mirrors.

I had to get honest with myself and with God and admit my sins. Anything that controls me or comes between God and me is an idol, and the first of God's Ten Commandments prohibits placing any other gods before Him.

I had made food a god. I had made being full a god. I had made the habit of having something in my mouth a god. I had made the feeling of satisfaction a god. Yet, like all false gods, the god of self-satisfaction is never satiated.

Same with me when it comes to food.

Who's in Control?

If you knew you were going to get a pink slip at work next week, especially in this tough economy, could you say, "It's not going to bother me. The Lord knows best"? That's what Paul said. If you're a student, how would you respond if your boyfriend ditched you? If you flunked a final exam? Could you still say, "God is in control. I trust Him"? The only way we can respond in such fashion is to take up our cross daily, follow Christ, and allow the Holy Spirit His rightful role of Controller and Guide.

My wife and I dated for years before marrying in our mid-30s. When we dated, I drove wherever we went and she sat in the passenger seat. We never had any problems with the arrangement. Now that we've been married a while, it's different.

The transformation started so slowly that at first I thought something was wrong with my car. I figured all the squeaking came from my worn engine belts. I'd hear, "Oooh, ooh, woooh, woooh, woooh." It sounded like a monkey.

The noise grew louder until I finally noticed Donna holding up her hands in front of the windshield, eyes wide open.

"What is wrong with you?" I asked.

She couldn't hold it any longer. She yelled a new warning every few moments: "Look out! Red light! Watch it! Look out for that car! You're too close to their bumper! Slow down!"

"What are you doing?" I yelled. "You're going to make me wreck!"

She didn't stop. At every curve or traffic light, Donna squeaked or yelled and stomped on her imaginary break pedal to no avail. She had no control of the car. I was the one at the wheel, no matter how much she sounded like a chimp.

When we reached the interstate, she complained I manipulated the accelerator too much, up and down, up and down, rocking her back and forth.

I shook my head. "It's on cruise control, for goodness sake."

Before long, she whined about feeling queasy: "Oh, you're making me car sick. Turn on the air. Please turn on the airrrrrrrrr" and buried her face in the air conditioner vent. Then she rolled down her window and hung her head out like a dog, tongue flapping in the wind.

Now if you come to our small town and see us in the car, Donna is at the wheel and I'm in the passenger seat mumbling and looking like a dork.

Our driving escapades mirror the Christian life. When we say, "Jesus, save me and come into my life," the Holy Spirit comes into our lives but we still are wrapped in flesh. We're not going to be perfect until we get to heaven. So we're going to face the same temptations we've always faced. We now have the power not to cave in to those temptations, but we're always going to hear the devil barking in our ears.

Not that I'm calling my wife the devil, but you know what I'm saying.

The more we allow the Holy Spirit to drive our lives, Satan can chirp all he wants but he doesn't have control anymore.

Paul makes another strong point in Philippians 3:19. He refers to the enemies of Christ "whose end is destruction, whose god is their belly, and whose glory is in their shame—who set their mind on earthly things."

When I struggled with my weight, I knew I was fat but my mind was so set on earthly things that I actually thought, "I'm not that fat, I'm still good looking." Addiction warps perception. But then I would see my photos and reality would set in again.

I was never more like the enemies of Christ, like a heathen, than when my appetites drove me and my god was my belly. I could've painted it gold and let people bow down to the Buddha.

Swallowing the truth means ignoring the obvious. It means allowing addiction to warp perception. Admitting the truth means accepting who's in charge.

Sid Bream is a friend of mine from college. He played first base for the Pittsburgh Pirates and Atlanta Braves and became famous for sliding safely into home to win the 1992 National League Championship Series and send the Braves to the World Series.

If Sid ever decided to take a break in the middle of a game and laid his mitt on first base and walked into the dugout, any ball hit to the right side of the infield would go directly to right field. Any ball hit anywhere else in the infield couldn't be thrown to first base for the out.

Sid actually had to place his hand in the mitt for it to function properly and for the game to flow correctly. He couldn't just place a thumb in the mitt and have it flop around on the end of his arm. Rather, he had to fill up that mitt with his hand to make it work right. The same is true with the Holy Spirit's work in our lives. We have to allow Him to fill us and control every single aspect of our existence.

This is why Paul, after describing the enemies of Christ whose god is their belly, describes those precious ones who belong to Jesus. Meditate on this beauty:

"But our citizenship is in heaven. And we eagerly await a Savior from there, the Lord Jesus Christ who, by the power that enables Him to bring everything under his *control*, will transform our lowly bodies so that they will be like his glorious body" (Philippians 3:20-21, NIV, *emphasis mine*).

My lowly body will be like His glorious body. Thank the Lord...

Same with me when it comes to food.

Chapter 4

MY BAD

"Enjoy the Freedom Fries"

The two paramedics stopped in their tracks when they got a load of me. I lay moaning on the couch in my living room. I wasn't married yet and lived on the family farm with my mother. To this day, I live in the same house I grew up in. At any moment I can walk into a room and smack dab into a flood of memories.

My bad back had flared up. It was about 1995 and I weighed about 280 pounds. I fluctuated among several different weights through the years. The pendulum swung from relatively healthy, as when I met Donna, to pleasantly plump and sometimes all the way to gross.

When I lay on the couch in severe back pain, I was stuck on gross.

I was in the middle of a tour and had to cancel all of my concerts for two months. My poor mother didn't know what to do. One day, the pain intensified and I couldn't budge an inch. We had to call 911. Due to my size and the pain, I called paramedics to the rescue.

The embarrassing part was that they didn't come to take me to the emergency room. They came to take me to a doctor's appointment. I couldn't make it to my family doctor any other way.

Thankfully, the ambulance didn't blare its sirens as it rumbled into my yard. They knew it was a non-emergency emergency. I heard the baritone of the engine and the swish of the air brakes as the burly paramedics scrambled to gather their effects and make their way inside.

When they walked in the door, my vision of "burly" vanished.

The paramedics were women. Little women.

The ladies walked in and stopped in their tracks when they saw this massive beached whale with a locked-up back and full bladder.

"Oh my," one of them said before she knew it. The other paramedic leaned toward her partner and whispered without turning her face.

"We might need some backup."

I wanted to crawl under a cushion. I've heard of police needing backup, but paramedics?

My dainty helpers dispensed with the required blood pressure and heart rate checks, asked me a few questions, and radioed the situation back to head-quarters. They didn't exactly have a walkie-talkie code for "lard-butt needs a lift," so they just said it—in a professional manner, of course.

"Um, yes, um, we're on location. Subject is incapacitated and is more than we can handle."

The radio squawked. "What's the problem?"

"We need more manpower, sir."

"More manpower? What do you mean?"

"Sir, we need assistance to lift him. He's a large individual."

"Can he not shift onto the gurney?"

"No, sir. He can't move on his own. Terrible back pain. We gotta have some muscle here."

Pause.

"Listen, we're, uh, we're—are you sure you can't move him?"

She was nodding before she pressed the button. "Positive."

Pause.

"10-4. Assistance on the way."

Right about then I would've signed Dr. Kevorkian's release if he wanted to help send me on to Jesus.

The wait seemed interminable before a fire truck full of men—burly men—wailed into the driveway. I guess they blared the siren because indeed no code existed for my predicament and for them it qualified as an emergency call. I was as red as their truck.

A few minutes later, they lifted and pushed the gurney into the ambu-lance, its legs folding underneath and jolting more pain throughout my back. It may have been the quickest completion of any assignment in Henry County Fire Department history.

The ambulance jostled toward the doctor's office, siren silent. The driver stopped at traffic lights and stop signs. It was a slow ride, an expensive but necessary lift into town.

Imagine that. I needed the dadgum fire department to lift me into an ambulance, and I needed a dadgum ambulance for a doctor's visit.

I've seen cable documentaries about morbidly obese people who couldn't move and whose rescuers tore down walls so forklifts could pick up the patients on their beds. I never envisioned I'd need a group of civil servants to help me make a doctor's visit.

Dr. Blissett had been my family doctor since I was kid. Every time he saw me in my adult years he told me to lose weight. He never failed to scold me. When we arrived at his office, the ambulance sat idling. Several moments passed. I didn't know what was going on and began to wonder whether Dr. Blissett was in the office. The paramedics didn't even bother trying to get me out of the ambulance because they knew they couldn't lift me back in.

Suddenly, the back doors swung open. There he stood, scowling at me.

"I told you!" he yelled. "This is ridiculous."

I don't think he said another word. He gave me some kind of painkiller on the spot so I could at least function and get to the bathroom. He whipped out his prescription pad and scribbled.

"Here," he said, snatching a sheet off the pad. "But you have to lose weight."

And he slammed the door.

Andy's Advice

Even the ambulance ride wasn't a wakeup call. My back eventually improved, but my physique and outlook didn't. Though I recognized I had a problem, though I admitted my addiction, though I was embarrassed by it, I still plowed into the buffet line.

The reason? For years I practiced one of the most prevalent Golden Nuggets: *Enjoy the Freedom Fries.*

That means I took liberty to eat anything I pleased and refused to accept responsibility for my actions. It's one thing to admit a problem, but it's quite another to own it.

I had to take personal responsibility for my habits by not passing the buck. It wasn't a glandular problem, it wasn't my grandmother's fault, and I wasn't gravitationally challenged. I didn't have a fat gene. I had a fat piece of bacon in my mouth.

If you want to stay fat or get even fatter, enjoy the freedom fries. They're crisp and salty and are crazy good with a cookies-and-cream milkshake, but in the end they clog up your heart in more ways than one. They block out common sense and offer a deceptive escape to only one kind of freedom, the freedom to choose to remain in a gut rut. They also block out communication with God. When you eat like I did, it's sin, and sin stymies communication with God. It's hard to hear a still small voice when you're scraping your plate.

I'm not a medical doctor or a scientist, but I know everyone is different and faces different challenges. I also know most people are experts at making excuses and passing the buck. In my case, I'd pass the buck and ask somebody to pass the mac-and-cheese.

I didn't see my weight as my responsibility. How could it be my responsibility since I was born this way? Since my mama made me clean my plate? Since I have a problem with metabolism? Since my daddy was fat too? It wasn't my fault, and since it wasn't my fault...*hey, are those brownies over there?*

The devil didn't make me reach for that appetizer either. I had to admit to myself I had a choice, and I learned a person chooses to eat to become what he is.

The movie *Shawshank Redemption* features several poignant moments, none more full of gravity than when lead characters Andy Dufresne and "Red" Redding sit in the prison courtyard with their backs against the cold block walls late in the movie. A resolute Andy has just emerged from a long turn in solitary confinement, and he does little more than stare and speak monotone through one last conversation with his buddy before escaping Shawshank prison. Red knows something is wrong. He protests Andy's desperate talk but can only listen as Andy spits out a line that still resonates with me.

"Comes down to a simple choice, really," Andy says. "Get busy livin' or get busy dyin'."

Every overweight person needs a Shawshank moment. We need to realize the sobering truth that every day we either get busy living or get busy dying. Our choices make or break us. People make time to do what they really want to do. If we really want to lose weight or eat healthy foods, we'll do it. When I really wanted to eat, I ate. Many nights, I lay on the couch until Donna fell asleep in the bedroom because I knew I could sneak out to eat and she wouldn't know it. Some people sneak out at night to see someone else. I snuck out to see burgers. I had a fling with the Dairy Queen.

I sacrificed sleep or work—and risked the possibility of a traffic ticket— to binge. Drive-thrus are open late, but some of my favorites close at 1 a.m.

Sometimes I had to wait on Donna to fall asleep so I could race to the restaurant before it closed. Johnny Law likes to cruise around at that hour looking either for drunks or addicts trying to score drugs. I was an addict, but by the time the cops got to me I'd have grease dripping off my chin.

I wasn't always big, so for me that was another strike against the "genealogical predisposition" excuse. Some people are big their entire lives. In elementary school I was thin. I have pictures of myself as a child when I looked almost gaunt. I grew bigger in junior high and high school, affecting everything, especially in high school. I enjoyed playing football and I was good at it because I could knock people backward off of the line of scrimmage, but I wasn't the good-looking football star. I was the kid whose mom bought his pants in the Husky section. That was one of my original embarrassing episodes.

When I reached college, I went for the hunk look. At least I tried.

I dated the same girl for three-and-a-half years at Liberty. One time she broke up with me, and I didn't say a word to anybody except my roommates. I fasted and prayed for five days. I didn't see her and didn't stalk her like I wanted. I stayed away. A week later she saw me after chapel and said, "Hey, whatcha doin'?" Wink, wink.

We got back together. But during that period, I worked like mad in the YMCA weight room, where I did bench presses, squats, situps, curls, shoulder presses, dead lifts, and various other torture techniques. I almost passed out as I lifted weights during my fast, but I stayed in shape.

One day I stepped on a set of scales and weighed 159. That stuck in my mind because I hit that weight only one time. I stayed in the 160s during that busy time period, but my average weight during college was 175. Then when I got out of college my weight started moving up to the 190s and higher.

All of which goes to prove my point.

I believe 99.9 percent of people can lose weight without surgery or pills or gimmicks—if they want to. I believe the Bible when it says these desperate cravings come from within. I also believe all of us have unique circumstances we face that can make the road to health easier or more difficult. Call it environment or upbringing, but it's another substantial factor in the equation.

Notice I didn't call it an excuse. I called it a factor. It's a reality, nonetheless, one that I know better than anyone because of the first time I saw an ambulance parked in the driveway of my farm home....

Ho Cakes and Frog Legs

Liberty College used a brilliant stroke of marketing during my senior year of high school. It sent a performance group to my school.

While their intentions were to evangelize, the performers left an incredible impression upon my young heart. One of their songs, "Love Them While You Can," became part of my own show years later. I remember one of the lead singers introducing the song by saying, "You need to go home tonight and tell your mom and dad you love them."

Charles Davis was larger than life in ways innumerable. He reached 280 pounds at his heaviest, a man's man with a barrel chest and a laugh that echoed. It never felt cool to go up to my 280-pound dad and put my arm around him and say, "Dad, I love you." So I never did. He was big into sports, especially football, which he made me play. In fact, he made me play every sport. I was pretty good at football. I wasn't good at basketball, but I played it. I was so bad that they created a new position for me on the basketball team: tailback. The coach looked at me and said, "Get your tail back on the bench."

Whatever the sport, my dad attended every game.

It was a Wednesday when the group from Liberty urged us to go home and tell our parents we loved them. I remember I went home and purposed in my heart to tell my dad I loved him. I don't know why, but I just…couldn't. I still don't know why.

The very next day, I was called to the school office. My brother waited on the other end of the phone line.

"You need to come home," he said. "Dad is not well." When I made it home, a fire truck and an ambulance sat in the driveway.

My dad died later that day.

I will always regret that I never took the opportunity to say, "I love you." He was fifty-seven years old when he died, and now that I'm forty-eight I realize how young he died. Doctors told us he had blood clots in his lungs, and every time he stood to his feet the blood clots moved. One eventually reached his heart and killed him. He had suffered from phlebitis, an inflammation of a vein that leads to blood clots, and wore a leg brace for some time.

My mother knew I loved her because I told her all the time. We didn't get along perfectly though. I learned to bicker by watching my parents, who fought just like other parents. Our frying pan was on a frequent flier program when I was kid. But I'm glad I told my mother I loved her because she died in my home in 2001.

Both of my parents were big people. Yet I'm convinced both could've lost weight if they wished. We just weren't conditioned to think that way. I grew up in an era when health wasn't on the forefront of society's consciousness. Instead, almost every meal was an event, and my mom excelled at it.

Her name was Geneva—Jean for short. She cooked big Southern meals, and my dad scarfed them down. Mashed potatoes and gravy, steaks, fried pork chops, and gooey macaroni and cheese. We counted helpings, not calories. My dad cleaned his plate every time. But then he would do something a lot of folks may find uncouth.

I watched him many a day as he rose from the table, took his clean plate to the sink, and then used his fork to eat out of the pots on the stove.

Dad loved food so much he experimented with it. He once made pancakes with beans mixed in just to see how it tasted. It was horrible. But he would try anything and loved all kinds of food.

My great-grandmother on my mother's side was 102 when she passed away. She never counted a fat gram, carbohydrate, or calorie. She never measured food. She certainly never dealt a stack of Deal-a-Meal cards. But, by golly, she ate biscuits and gravy every day. She made a bunch of regular biscuits but saved enough dough for one big one. She called it a Ho Cake.

I've told that story in Vermont and they looked at me like, "Huh? Ho Cake? What is that?"

It's a biscuit on steroids, a flat one with a good crust. My great-grandmother would cover the Ho Cake with sorghum syrup and mix it up on the plate, then wash it down with an ice cold glass of milk. We called it "Good Vitamin D Milk" back then. At supper time, she ate green beans with fatback in it. She ate like this and yet lived until she was 102. Her daughter passed away at 94.

Farm life revolves around food. Most of the time, you're simply raising your keep, whether it's livestock or crops. We had both.

I had a pet pig as a kid, and we ate him later. How's that for loving food? Poor fellow limped around the pen as we worked on him one leg at a time. I mean, he was a pet. We didn't have the heart to eat him all at once.

I don't remember his name, but I remember shooting and cleaning him. My dad tried to teach me how to kill a chicken so we could eat the thing, but I couldn't ever figure out how to ring a chicken's neck.

Few varmints were off-limits, and we didn't kill anything we didn't eat. We went squirrel hunting, and my neighbors taught me how to make rabbit boxes so we could catch rabbits for a good meal. We killed and cleaned turtle and my mother made turtle soup. We had frog legs. We floated onto our little lake in an aluminum boat at night and used a huge beam of light to shine back toward the banks. When we saw two beady little eyes staring back at us we pointed right between those eyes with a .22 rifle and scrounged up some supper. The bigger the frog, the meatier the leg. Tastes like chicken.

Every year, my dad tended a large garden. One of the reasons I don't maintain a garden now is the emotional scar I carry from my childhood garden. On Saturday mornings when most kids watched cartoons and played, I had to hoe the garden or pick okra. I remember one Saturday morning I was on the phone with a girl from school. My dad said, "C'mon, we've got to go work in the garden."

"OK, be there in a minute." I kept talking on the phone.

"C'mon, we've got to go," he said.

"OK, just a sec."

I kept on talking. He called out again. I kept talking.

A few minutes later, the door to my bedroom swung open. He whipped out his knife. I felt my eyes widen. Suddenly I wasn't talking any more. He grabbed the phone line extending from the wall and cut it.

"I told you to come on," he said.

I was in the garden in a matter of seconds. And I had to fix the phone myself.

Charles Davis was serious about his food. Yet I was just getting started when it came to learning bad eating habits.

Too Young

Liberty College introduced me to a whole new world of eating—literally.

Not long after I reached campus, a friend wanted to try out for SMITE—a group of traveling singers like the one that performed at my high school—and he asked me to go with him.

I relented only because I was a homesick freshman eight hours away from Stockbridge. I needed something to pass the time. I'd call home and whimper, "Mama, I want to come home."

Dad already had passed away and she had no one to back her but she still said, "You're not coming home because I'm not losing my deposit."

After the first round of SMITE tryouts, they handed us the words to "God is So Good." A lot of the candidates were big-time music majors and well-known performers on campus. At the time, I had no idea who they were and didn't care.

I sang and apparently did well but I still didn't care. I probably did well because I didn't care. I didn't feel the slightest pressure. I just walked onstage and wailed away.

As I made the early rounds of cuts, much like an early version of *American Idol*, I realized I should take it more seriously because a scholarship hung in the balance. At one of the final cuts, we had to sing in front of everybody—including all of my competitors and other students from past SMITE teams. We sang "God is So Good" again. The piano guy started the song and I belted it. This time, something wasn't right. Piano Man stopped after a few moments.

"Let's try that in a different key," he said. That was the polite way to tell me I stunk.

We switched the key and I sang OK. A guy already on the team saddled up next to me afterward.

"I'm not supposed to tell you this," he said. "You didn't do so well that time, but Roscoe Brewer really likes you." Then I felt the nerves. Roscoe was the big cheese, one of Dr. Falwell's top lieutenants.

Out of 160 candidates, I was one of fifteen people named to the team and awarded a full scholarship for the rest of my college career. I had a strange mixture of emotions. I celebrated doing well, but deep down I did not want to be a part of a missions group that traveled overseas. I sat there after hearing the great news and it dawned on me that in a matter of months I would be headed to Brazil. I didn't want to go to Brazil. I wanted to go back home to Georgia.

My tune soon changed for one reason. Food.

Not only did I earn a full scholarship to Liberty and the privilege of traveling around the world, but I also got to eat like crazy. Within two weeks after I made the team, they said, "We're going to introduce you to the world."

Fresh from my tiny hometown in the Deep South, I found myself in the middle of Manhattan in a matter of weeks. We spent a week and a half in New York City, the melting pot of the world. They took us all over the five boroughs to meet people of different ethnicities and to introduce us to various cultures and foods. We also witnessed to people on the street. It served as an introduction and training session for our group—and for me when it came to food. It was a delicious time. I count it a blessing in many ways, but I also look back and realize it helped set into motion some destructive appetites and habits.

In the first weeks of real freedom in my young life, I began making choices that conditioned me to overeat.

Brazil had unbelievable steakhouses. If you've ever tried a Brazilian steakhouse like Fogo de Chao here in the States, you understand. In Brazil back then, an all-you-can-eat meal at a steakhouse cost only five dollars. Today, it's still only about seven bucks.

I'd look like the Michelin Man if I lived in Brazil. The coroner's report would read, "Death by meat."

I went to Korea and tried the Kim-chi (fermented vegetables). I went to South Africa and ate anything they put in front of me. At one Asian Indian restaurant, I loved the food even when it was so spicy hot few others would touch it. One skinny guy in our group walked out looking like he had a tumor on his ankle. I looked down at his foot as he walked a little stiff-legged.

I pointed at the bulge on his ankle. "You OK?" I asked.

He nodded and smiled. Then he pulled off his shoe and sock. He had stuffed all his hot rice into his sock because he didn't want to offend our hosts. He had finished with the only clean plate in the joint, and they had doted over him. My mouth and stomach were on fire, but I still laughed at his Curry Fried Ankle.

In American Samoa, the locals conducted a traditional tribal night and cooked a whole pig for us, head and all. I think it still had some hair on the carcass when they served it. Most of our group turned up their noses. I just cut around the hair and gnawed away.

They passed around half a coconut filled with a passion fruit concoction. I was known on the team as the guy who would try anything. *Give it to Scott.* It was like the old Life Cereal commercial: "Give it to Mikey. He'll try anything. Hey Mikey!"

I'd never had a bad meal in my life—until then. In American Samoa I tried tofu and it tasted like a sponge.

I now know all of this played into my food addiction. That may sound like a rationalization, but I think it's a reality. I know my struggles with weight and food were more a product of environment and personal choices than they were genetics. I had a problem with a Jean all right, and she could fry up a mess of pork chops.

More often than not, we are the sum of our individual decisions. That's scary stuff, but the Bible backs it up.

In Proverbs 23:7, wise King Solomon states that a man behaves like he thinks. I like the King James translation: "For as he thinketh in his heart, so is he." Even if what we believe about ourselves is not true, our behavior will reflect our belief in that lie. The Bible says Satan is the father of lies, and he uses lies to deceive us into believing wrong thoughts about ourselves, other people, and many other subjects. The Bible also says he comes to steal, kill, and destroy. At the same time, it says he disguises himself as an angel of light.

> More often than not, we are the sum of our individual decisions.

He can make everything sound amazing, including food. He can make mundane menus appealing. He can make commercials so appetizing we can almost smell them.

And every bit of it is designed to steal our joy, kill our hope, and destroy us all together.

Satan knows his deceptions are effective because we're no different than his first victims. Those of us who struggle with weight control have no trouble understanding why Adam and Eve suffered The Fall over food. Now, obviously, the fruit from the tree of the knowledge of good and evil was merely the object that revealed hearts already tilted away from God. From the very beginning, the enemy of our souls has pursued one basic deception: He wants us to believe that anything other than God will fulfill us. Is it not telling that our first stumbling block in this area—the first thing Satan used to draw out our self-centered desires from deep within us—was food?

'Course, if it had been an Oreo tree, I would've busted hell wide open in the first two minutes.

The same desire that came from within Eve to drive her to pluck off the one fruit she wasn't supposed to eat is the same desire that makes you and me reach out in a repeated, mindless, habitual, indulgent fashion to gorge ourselves.

That's why we can't say the devil made us do it. We do it to ourselves. It comes from within. Adam and Eve didn't have to order the Good-and-Evil Blue Plate Special that day, and I don't have to pull out of Taco Bell with a greasy-bottomed sack at 12:56 a.m.

Wise King Solomon also said, "Keep your heart with all diligence, for out of it spring the issues of life" (Proverbs 4:23, NKJV). That is one of the most well-known verses in the Bible. I'm ashamed to say it's so familiar I zip past it. Now read the next line.

"Put away from you a deceitful mouth, and put perverse lips far from you." *Ouch.*

I've read that many times without thinking about it in the context of food. Its primary warning is toward speech, but it is not a stretch to ascribe the same truth to eating. My watering mouth can deceive me so easily, and my old eating habits were nothing if not perverse.

In the same way, Proverbs 13:3 draws a bullseye on my little dieting heart:

> *"He who guards his mouth preserves his life, but he who opens wide his lips shall have destruction."*

I think I'll write that verse in calligraphy and use a QWLCA magnet to stick it on my refrigerator door. I wish someone had read Proverbs to me while I was globetrotting with SMITE. Instead, I had to learn these truths the hard way.

As Dr. Blissett would say, my weight problem was my fault. It wasn't a glandular problem. It wasn't because someone was too harsh to me in second grade. And it wasn't even heredity, unless you consider learning the bad habits of parents heredity.

No, my weight problem came one bite at time. And to prove it, those Proverbs say a mouthful.

Part of my wanting to lose weight now is because I didn't want to end up like my father, dead at the age of 57. Toward the end of my fat years, Donna looked at me one day and said, "Don't you want to be around for Dylan?" He's our six-year-old grandson. Before he was born, people asked us what we wanted to be called as grandparents, and I said, "Big Daddy." My dad was called Big Daddy. That's what Dylan calls me.

My personal doctor now is a Korean fellow in his 70s. He's a great guy, but he needs to work on his bedside manner.

I met him about a year before I began the QWLCA program. I had never laid eyes on the man, but I waited in one of his exam rooms, all 300 pounds lapped over a little table. In walked Dr. Kim. He didn't say my name. He didn't say hello. And he didn't smile. He opened the door, stopped in his tracks when he saw me, and asked one question in his clipped English.

"You ever hear Weight Watchers?"

That's the first thing my new doctor said to me. It stung, and it was rude, but, like Dr. Blissett before him, Dr. Kim tried to get my attention.

"You too young. You too young to be this big," he said. "You can do it if you try. You can do it."

Indeed, I was the *only* one who could do it.

While they were only trying to help, it didn't matter what Donna and the doctors said. It didn't matter that firemen had to lift me into an ambulance for a doctor's visit. It didn't even matter how many bad habits I picked up from my family and from traveling the world.

What mattered is that I accepted responsibility for my food addiction. I had to sign my name to it before I was liable for it. To escape it, I had to own it.

I visited Dr. Kim after my huge weight loss. He was elated because he felt like his little lecture helped, which it did. He asked me to write down everything I had done to lose weight so he could share it with his other patients who tell him they can't lose weight.

"I want to hand it to them and say, 'Yes, you can. Read this,'" he said.

He was satisfied when I told him I was writing a book about it. He asked for copies for his patients.

"Maybe we can take a photograph of us together," I said. "We'll put it in the book so everyone will know who the doctor is who blurted out that I needed to be on Weight Watchers."

He nodded and smiled. I saw his wheels turning, but this time he bit his tongue. Maybe it was my imagination, but I could tell he was thinking of the photograph and wanted to give me another zinger:

"At least now you don't need wide-angle lens."

Chapter 5

REVELATION

"Welcome to the Waffle House"

Fat folks know some things better than thin folks. We know just how deep the pink marks can go from being corded by underwear. We know what tastes good. And we know, better than most, just how important oxygen is. I got so fat that at times I could barely breathe. When it comes to living, air helps.

This is why a big belly and sleeping don't go together. It seemed as if the bigger I got, the sleepier I got.

At my heaviest, I lived in the lazy man's vicious cycle: Stay up half the night when no one else is around so you can stuff your gut as you please, and then sleep too long, lose valuable daylight and productivity, and set up yourself to repeat the same undisciplined regimen the next day.

I still have scars from the double-edged sword of being my own boss. For an addict, it can mean having too much freedom. And in some ways how I make my living helped me gloss over my issues rather than address them.

Comedy was my cheat sheet on life. It was my mask, my fantasy to escape reality. Deep inside, I felt bad not only physically but also emotionally, psychologically, and spiritually. I grew depressed. I was tired and broken down. I was pathetic. Yet I always turned to my humor, my "ministry" of making people laugh. Truth is, it ministered to me more than anyone. Making people laugh made me feel good and lent me worth, at least while I was onstage. It made me feel better if I could make someone else feel better, as if I'd accomplished something. To that end, I guess God used me in spite of myself.

But while everybody laughed, my vicious cycle continued.

My niece, Ashley, worked in my home office for several years, helping me book and coordinate my concerts and various chores. I had one ironclad rule for her.

"If anyone calls before 10 a.m. and wonders where I am," I said, "Just tell them I'm in the word."

That didn't mean I'd squirreled myself away somewhere to study the Bible. I nicknamed my bed "the word."

It was an off-hand comment I made a few times, and I didn't think it was that funny. But Mark Lowry cackled hard when he heard it. He called me one night at about 11 p.m. He knew I'd be parked in front of the television.

"Man, my concert was sold out tonight, just packed," he said. "They loved 'the word' story."

"Mark! You used my line?"

"Yeah, they loved it," he said. "I'll tell you what, I'll pay you for that joke."

Mark honored his word and paid me every month for a year to help him write. I've still got the contract somewhere. It's strange, but I don't consider myself a stand-up comedian who tells jokes. Most of my humor comes out of life experiences. I began coming up with funny stories for Mark, and he used some and didn't use others. I helped Mark with his newsletter each month, reviewing it before publication. I made notes of funny items and suggested edits or additions. He wrote it, but I added spice.

"I just supported you is what I did," he joked on the phone one time. "Like a missionary."

I remember sitting in a room at Word Records with Mark, Martha Bolton, Cory Edwards, and Bubba Smith. Cory wrote the animated movies *Hoodwinked* and *Hoodwinked Too*. We'd sit around a big conference room table and throw out ideas for Mark's next comedy video, one of the most invigorating ways of constructing comedy.

Several of Mark's videos have gone gold in sales, and I appear in all but a few of them. We always played off of my size. In one video, I play Big Judd Brown. I wear a shirt sprayed down with water to make me appear soaked in sweat. I look horrible, perfect for a skit themed as "Big Judd Brown: You Never Get a Second Chance to Make a First Impression."

The video *Remotely Controlled* centers upon Mark watching TV while on his tour bus. It shows him watching his own comedy routine but he grows bored with it and changes channels. They're all fake, obviously, but he lands on a channel on which the announcer blares, "Two beautiful women who love the same man, and that man is UGLY." The camera focuses on me. I sit on a couch with a big cigar hanging out of my mouth and two gorgeous girls—I have no idea where they found them—on either side of me. They fight over me. It looks like something off of a silly reality show, which is ironic because scenes like two beautiful women fighting over a disgustingly fat guy are more fantasy than reality.

In the past, a lot of my comedy routine featured my stories of growing up on a farm. I usually ran my jokes by Mark first.

He'd laugh and say, "You need to put that in your show. That's funny." So I did. Even now, most of my stories come out of painful moments or arguments with my wife. Not that we're going to divorce, but everybody has issues. As Dr. Falwell used to say, divorce is never an option. Murder maybe, but never divorce. I try to look at the funny side of our squabbles and tell the tales. Here's a true story:

Donna woke up angry at me the other day. Have you ever had your spouse do this to you? When she awoke, she was mad at me because I wronged her in a dream. She stayed mad for the first half of the day. I had to leave the house for a while. And it was *dream*.

Telling stories out of life meant telling stories about my girth, but much of the fat humor covered my embarrassment. Instead of ignoring it and climbing under a rock, I thought, "I'm just going to get it out there, make a joke out of it, and get past it." That was my way of dealing with it in public.

How ironic that I could do it in public but struggled so mightily to confront myself personally.

That's a sign of a true addict, though. Put on a show. Act like life is grand.

Ignore the obvious.

Laugh to Keep from Crying

Humor often comes out of tragedy. Some of the most famous comedians in history laughed at themselves to keep from crying. Former *Saturday Night Live* actor Chris Farley was one of the most hilarious comics I've ever seen. Yet I suspect at least some of his humor masked the pain he felt over his weight. Think about it. One of his most famous skits featured Patrick Swayze and Farley as male dancers. Swayze was convincing in the part because of his physique. Farley flailed in front of an entire nation on live TV, his hairy gut hanging out. The only way you can do that is to block out the shame, go the opposite direction, and get wild and crazy. It lets people laugh but it means opening yourself to intense scrutiny, and that is a scary place.

The downside to that scenario can be deflating. Perhaps not every big person experiences this, but for me relationships could be minefields. It seemed at times that people liked me when I made them laugh. When I wanted to be myself, the picture changed. It seemed nobody cared to be around me. Maybe it wasn't reality. Maybe it was just how I felt. When I weighed 309 pounds, it was easy to make people laugh when I joked about myself. But when it came time to be serious or deal with a relationship or talk about something personal, the reaction seemed to be more like, "Ohhh. He's so pathetic. I don't want to be around this."

That's the reason I kept making people laugh. I had to ensure people liked me—all of me. Much of the material I'm developing now has nothing to do with being big. I'm discovering life has other funny subjects. But just as my baggy clothes draped my physical body, a lot of my old comedy draped my soul.

> That's the reason I kept making people laugh. I had to ensure people liked me—all of me.

Using comedy as a mask was therapeutic in one way, but it also worked against me. Why change my eating habits when being fat provided the primary fodder for my livelihood? Losing weight meant losing a huge chunk of my comedy routine.

I stayed stuck in neutral for a long time. I knew I was obese. I knew it was my fault. I even knew it was sin. I just chose not to choose to do anything about it, and that bogged me in the mire of my next Golden Nugget: *Welcome to Waffle House.*

True Southerners smirk with skewed pride in our Waffle Houses. The restaurant chain has something of a cult following. Most of the cult members wear size XL, but at least they're faithful. Places like Waffle House make it hard for big folks to make up their minds to do something about their weight. The food is just too good.

But the word *waffle* is more dangerous to a fat person as a verb than as a noun.

If you want to stay fat or get even fatter, keep waffling in the same status quo. No need to put any thought into what you eat—or how much or when or whether it's dead or alive. Just keep chewing the same fat, saying the same lame lies to yourself over and over. Refuse to get better. Let your mind wander the buffet of life. Indulge your food fantasies. Continue being large and less than you can be.

I know it so well because I lived there so long.

I hated being stuck at this stage. It felt like jail and yet I held the key all the while. Come to think of it, that's part of the punishment. I couldn't make up my mind to do something about the status quo even though my quo was sickeningly large. While this step is the catalyst to regaining control over weight, it also happens to be the toughest aspect of losing weight.

People ask me everywhere I go, "What made you stick with this diet?" That is the foremost question I face, and for good reason. Everybody, and I mean every single overweight person who's ever strained to button his jeans, has struggled to make up his mind to do something about his waistline and then stick with it.

So, what gives? How do we make up our minds not just to lose weight but also to lose weight permanently and forge a forever kind of change? I don't know if it's possible to pinpoint a one-size-fits-all answer. It's different for each person. For the longest time, I couldn't offer a viable answer even for myself.

It's reflexive to blurt out a canned response like, "I don't know. I guess I just wanted to get healthy." Well, duh. Everyone wants to be healthy.

I had dozens of motivations to lose weight, some of which I share in the rest of this chapter. But what flipped my switch for the last time?

To be honest, I didn't know my answer until I sat down to write this book.

Counting

Walking around in a Serotonin-induced haze is not my idea of fun. I used to stay so drowsy that I'd nod off in a car wash. Then I found out one of the reasons for the constant fog. It's called sleep apnea, and it's a condition in which a person intermittently stops breathing during sleep. The lack of oxygen diminishes restful sleep and leaves the person tired throughout the day. I didn't realize I had it until my wife told me.

One morning, before the period in which Donna banished me to the guest bedroom to sleep, I awoke gasping for air sometime around 3 a.m.

Donna stared at me and looked at the watch in her hand.

"You went a minute and a half and didn't breathe," she said.

"Well, when were you going to poke me?" I said, squinting to bring her into focus. "Two minutes? Five minutes? When I turned blue?"

She started shaking her head and tried to speak but I cut her off.

"I mean, is there a point where you finally say, 'Well, I wonder if he's going to keep breathing'?"

I have a friend who's a big person who sleeps with an apnea machine. It blows a constant stream of air through a hose and into a mask worn over the face. It's called a Continuous Positive Airway Pressure (CPAP) machine. My buddy recently told me he had an appointment with a clinic to undergo another sleep test as a checkup. I told him the story about Donna counting how long I went without breathing without nudging me awake.

"Yeah, she was counting, all right," he said. "She was counting $100,000, $200,000, $300,000 in life insurance money."

Those years were difficult. I sometimes awoke gasping for air. Though I never underwent testing for apnea I did try a CPAP machine. A friend got a new machine and let me borrow his old one. This move isn't exactly approved by the American Medical Association, so don't try it at home. I never could get the thing to help me because I would wake up, mouth wide open and as dry as a cotton boll in a drought. Even asleep my biggest problem was opening my mouth.

I should've picked up on the fact that I wasn't breathing in my sleep long before Donna had fun with her little counting game. According to the materials I read, I had all the tell-tale signs of apnea:

Fatigue? Yep, I could check that one on the list.

Significant daytime drowsiness? Check.

Snoring? Double check.

My body has a snoring threshold at 220 pounds. When I reached that weight, I apparently had grown enough fat inside my nasal passages that they began flapping whenever I conked out. The heavier I got, the bigger they got, and the more they flapped. When I topped 300 pounds, those suckers flapped so hard they sounded like a moose call. It got to the point where I began waking myself with my own snoring. I tried everything to quit snoring, but the moose kept moaning.

I sometimes roomed with Mark Lowry when I accompanied him on some of his tours. He'd sleep on one bed and I'd sleep on the other. One night, my snoring woke him.

"Scott! Scott!"

"Huh?"

"You're snoring. Uh-uh. Ain't happening. It's worth getting you a whole 'nother room." Now he sounded like my wife. From then on, he paid for another room.

At other times, I've had road managers travel with me on my own tours. One guy, Billy (not Billy Lord), roomed with me. After we ate supper and returned to the hotel room, I conked out on my bed. I woke up at about 3 a.m. and looked over only to see a mattress with no sheets. Nothing was on his Billy's bed. No covers. No pillows. No Billy. Where did he go?

It wasn't the Rapture because I knew I was more spiritual than that dude. I got up and looked around the room and then stumbled to the bathroom. I opened the door and looked down. There he was, curled up on a makeshift pallet in the tub.

He looked up, one eye closed. "Man, you snore!"

I'm cheap but I'm also compassionate. I started paying for an extra room so my staff could be rested enough to help me.

I've seen people snoring on airplanes and thought, "Oh, Lord, please don't ever let that be me." I like to book an aisle seat to enjoy the extra room. When I was big, I went to sleep fast but awoke with bruises. I rubbed and looked up in time to see Flight Attendant Barbie smile and wave "Buh-bye" after cramming the beverage cart into the half of my body that stuck out in the aisle. One day I worked up the gumption to ask my road manager if I snored on the plane. To my relief, he said I didn't. When I slept sitting up, I was quiet.

In my fat days, I sometimes hassled for breath as my gut compressed my diaphragm like a concrete block on a balloon. I struggled with simple chores like walking to the mailbox (all joking aside, I had a hard time with this), taking out the trash, or climbing steps.

Now that I've lost weight, I literally breathe easier and don't snore at all. I've abandoned the guest bedroom and reclaimed my spot next to my wife on the right side of our bed. I no longer keep her awake with my snoring or body heat—or with the temptation to play her little counting game when my chest doesn't move.

Sanctuary

My rumble through the airport detailed in Chapter One embarrassed me, as did the episodes in which I broke the toilet seat and two different beds and needed an ambulance for a doctor's visit.

Those moments turned my face red, for sure, but personal humiliation is different. It carries a different weight. As I describe some of these instances, please understand I'm being transparent not to demonstrate how pathetic I was or to elicit sympathy. No one had to tell me I was pathetic, and I didn't deserve sympathy because I brought my grief on myself.

Instead, I share these personal humiliations to detail the many reasons I almost didn't have a choice but to do something about my weight. Plus, I pray my honesty comforts others in similar situations and lets them know the depths from which anyone is capable of emerging.

I realized how nasty obese I had grown when I could no longer wear shoes with laces. I literally could not reach over to tie shoes. When I tried, I'd lose my breath or have to catch myself before falling over. I switched to slip-on shoes.

> I realized how nasty obese I had grown when I could no longer wear shoes with laces.

Other sickening side effects surfaced in the bathroom.

I can't tell you how important my daily toilet time is to me. Maybe that sounds weird, but my bathroom is a bit of a sanctuary. The bathroom is where I read a great deal. It's where I think. I come up with funny stories. It's my personal retreat. At one point, I even had a television in the bathroom so I could camp out as long as I liked. When you don't get married until your mid-30s, you become a bit set in your ways and guard your space. My space happens to flush with blue water.

Imagine, then, the sobering reality that my butt had grown so large I had to buy the largest toilet seat I could find. I couldn't even use the guest bathroom toilet anymore because it was the old-fashioned, smaller kind and my butt wouldn't fit on it. I felt like was sitting on a thimble.

The shower presented another hazard. When a remodeling project on our main bathroom bogged down, I had to use the guest bathroom's tiny modular shower. It was about four feet square. I didn't step in and get stuck, but I came close. It was great for cleaning though. I just lathered up real good and turned around a few times to take care of all four walls at once. *Scrubbing bubbles, scrubbing bubbles, hoo-hoo-hoo-hoo!*

Even more fallout emerged in the bedroom.

In my ever-fluctuating battle, I had lost a good bit of weight before I met Donna. I started gaining after we married in December 1998. Over time, my weight gain affected even the physical part of our marriage. Donna told me while we were dating (and I was smaller) that if she had met me when I was as big as my video character Big Judd Brown she never would have dated me. I don't blame her. I would feel the same way about her. I don't mean to be ungodly, but I like somebody who looks decent. Perhaps that's shallow and hypocritical, but I'm being bone honest.

As I got bigger—250 pounds, then 260, then 270 and the scales groaned ever higher—our sex life suffered. What was appealing about me? Sex is physical and involves physical attraction. It wasn't exactly a romance-novel moment when I looked over, wiggled my eyebrows, and asked, "Hey, baby, wanna have some fun?" My form of birth control was getting undressed with the lights on.

Then again, dressing myself was like enduring an obstacle course.

I hated buying clothes. I shopped at Wal-Mart most of the time and purchased big jeans and big shirts and left them untucked long before it was stylish. I didn't want to be the guy who tucked in his shirt but had his gut hanging over his beltline for all to see.

We all have different body types. Some people have fat legs, some have big guts, rear ends, or chests. I had a huge gut with normal legs. My waist was so large that I had to have extra-large pants, which meant the pants legs dwarfed my skinny legs. I looked dumpy. I had a picture in mind of what I was supposed to look like as I got dressed, and then I'd look in the mirror and think, "Oh, I don't look anything like I thought. Awful. Just awful."

I don't know why I had that thought process. Maybe it's because I was thin before I got fat, but the mirror doesn't lie.

Neither does my wife.

I would dress in one of my big, drape-like shirts, turn to Donna and ask, "Honey, does this make me look fat?" Yes, even men use that line. Donna would roll her eyes at me.

"No, that shirt doesn't make you look fat. Your face makes you look fat.

Your gut makes you look fat. Your fat makes you look fat. Are you kidding me?"

Actually, she never said that, but her look did.

I guess the proper question would have been, "Does this make me look less fat than I really am?" I tried to use clothes to minimize my body and hide from my true appearance. I don't think it ever worked.

Black clothing is supposed to be slimming. I wore black clothes all the time. One of my friends looked at me and shook his head. "You need something darker."

I knew I was in trouble then. Goth isn't in when you're middle-aged.

Yet another frustration occurred before Jerry Falwell's funeral. I had to purchase a suit at Casual Male XL, where professional athletes shop. I needed a size 52 suit. That's 12 sizes larger than my college suit from Hong Kong.

All of these little moments coalesced into an unmistakable and constant urge to change. Yet none had the impact as one fitful and faith-filled shortcoming that rocked me to my core. I finally had to hold up a mirror not to ask what I saw....

But what God saw.

Before and After

Anytime I see an advertisement for the latest diet or exercise fad, I never trust the Before-and-After photos. I'm convinced some of them show two different people. Here's Tubby before. Here's Thomas afterward. Perhaps Tubby and Thomas are brothers separated at birth, but they ain't the same dude.

In other ads, a grainy candid photo shows a big lady at a family reunion, mouth full of egg salad and wearing something that looks like either a maternity blouse or a hot air balloon. In the next photo, somebody who doesn't come close to resembling Reunion Girl postures in spandex shorts and a sports bra, abs ripped. And she did it in six weeks.

Other examples include photos clearly of the same man, but in the Before photo he's a little meaty and in the After photo he's sucking his gut in so far his navel touches his spine. I have a rule of thumb: Don't trust the photo if you can see someone's entire bottom rib.

You can't always believe the Before and After.

I believe appearance is important for a lot of reasons. The Bible says to give no appearance of evil. I gave the appearance of pound cake. The truth of what I'm about to share with you is proven every week at my concerts now. Now that I've lost weight and look less sloppy and at least presentable, more people attend. Whether it's right or wrong, my audiences are larger now that I'm smaller.

Even my mother, who was a big woman, fell victim to this thinking. She called out from her bedroom one time.

"Turn it on the Christian station. Who is that playing?" I changed channels to see whom she was watching.

"That's Michael W. Smith," I said.

"Hmm," she said almost under her breath. "He's good-looking."

While I believe God is blessing my obedience in taking care of His temple, I also believe in human nature, and humans are shallow. A third of Carman's audience came to see him because he's good-looking. We can debate the morality of the phenomenon, but the truth is that his looks attracted people. Not that I'm good-looking now, but at least I don't look like Shamu anymore.

Of all the motivations to lose weight through the years, I can point to two that most helped me escape the waffling stage. The first came during the middle of one of my concerts.

Premier Productions is one of the larger Christian production companies. They've promoted everyone from Casting Crowns to Toby Mac to the Comedy Bus Tour, which I've been a part of for INO Records. A few years ago, Premier produced a big comedy concert featuring three comedians. Actually, it was two comedians and me. That was the night I realized who I was—or at least who I wasn't.

We were in Fort Wayne, Indiana, and each of us performed 20-minute segments before an intermission followed by separate 10-minute finales. In the middle of all the laughter and showmanship, I had a revelation.

Most places hire me as a comedian and promote me as a comedian. But that night in Fort Wayne, I realized I'm not a comedian. When I started out at Liberty, I was a singer on scholarship for music. I wanted to be a singer. My friends are singers. Mark Lowry started out as a singer. He doesn't like to be called a comedian either. He prefers to be called a humorist because he tells stories, not jokes.

I started out in the same world, performing as a singer who also spoke at revivals. My main spiritual gift is evangelism, and I see myself as an evangelist. That's the reason I conduct Christian school conferences, where we see a lot of kids come to know Christ. Every concert I perform, even though it's a comedy concert, I present the Gospel and see people surrender their lives to Christ every week. That's my heart and passion.

I walked onstage that night in Fort Wayne and watched another guy close out the show. He's a great guy and a great friend, but I left feeling flat when he closed by saying, "It's been a great night. Live for God. Love Jesus. Goodnight."

I just stared at the crowd filing out.

"Man. We have a huge audience," I thought. "Let's just share the Gospel real quick." It was a great night. There's nothing wrong with making people laugh and having a little fun with comedy. But it hit me like never before that comedy is not what I'm called to do. I'm called to preach the Gospel, and comedy is just a tool.

> I spoke one thing with my mouth but proved with my gut that I kept Jesus reserved for certain compartments of my life but not for all of me.

I returned home, wheels turning. If I'm called as an evangelist and nothing is more important than people's souls and eternal destiny, then how could I ask them to take me seriously when I stood before them to talk about the Savior who rescues us from all of our sins and burdens? My massive burden had a belly button and lapped over my belt. I spoke one thing with my mouth but proved with my gut that I kept Jesus reserved for certain compartments of my life but not for all of me.

Grappling with this healthy dose of conviction nudged me closer and closer to a watershed moment.

Romans 12:1-2 became something of a battle cry for me. In it, Paul addresses the church in Rome, a city so known for hedonism, debauchery, and indulgence of all fleshly appetites that the Apostle Peter refers to it as "Babylon." Paul encourages believers not to be conformed to this world but to be transformed by the renewing of our minds. The way our minds are transformed is through the washing of the water of the Word—studying the Bible and obeying what it says.

Those familiar with this passage often focus on the first half of Romans 12:2, which is Paul's admonition not to be conformed to the world but to be transformed by renewing our minds. For me, a man struggling with the impact my appearance had on my testimony, the Before-and-After sections of this verse brought the message home full force.

Before the famous Verse 2, Paul says in Verse 1, "I beseech you therefore, brethren, by the mercies of God, that you present your bodies a living sacrifice, holy, acceptable to God." I know God's altar is big, but I needed more than my fair share of space to present my body a living sacrifice. I'm sure you've heard people say they "just want to sit at the feet of Jesus" in Bible study and prayer. That was an issue for me. I needed His help to get back up.

The second half of Verse 2—the *After* portion—is just as powerful. Paul says God wants us not to conform to the world and to allow the Lord to transform our minds for one reason: "that you may prove what is that good and acceptable and perfect will of God."

Standing offstage in Fort Wayne, I knew I wanted to prove God's good, acceptable, and perfect will to a watching world that longs to see authentic faith lived out loud. I knew the Before-and-After snapshots of Romans 12:1-2 had to rule my life.

The second of my two main motivations for lasting life change was a realization that didn't register in my conscious mind until I started writing this book.

It dawned on me that it was more work to stay fat than it was to lose weight.

That's what broke the dam for me. The little embarrassments were bad. The spiritual conviction was worse. But the lifestyle, living as an obese man, was debilitating. I've made it clear that I'm lazy, but I'm too lazy even to stay fat. It was just too difficult. Life had become untenable.

It took an incredible amount of energy and time to arrange my day around the number of meals and snacks required to maintain the number of calories my body grew acclimated to consuming. I thought only of food, and it drained me.

I was sick and tired of being sick and tired. I wasn't scared of dying. I thought I might die sooner than I should, and I probably would have. After thinking through this book, I know I decided to change because I grew miserable and exhausted not just from carrying the weight but also from maintaining it.

I threw up my flabby arms and said, "That's it. I can't do this anymore."

Everything was work. It was work to get dressed. It was work to tie shoes or to walk anywhere. It was work to wiggle into the car and fetch another sack of burgers. I don't want this book to sound pathetic, but I was pathetic at that point. I could joke about it in my routine, and part of it was funny to a degree. But when you pass the 300 mark and keep going, it ain't funny anymore.

If you've reached that point, or if you fear reaching that point, then let me save you a lot of heartache, trouble, and money. It took years of little motivations to add up to a few big motivations before I stopped waffling and overcame the psychological barricade that losing weight is too hard. To the contrary, I had to work harder to stay big, and I found losing 132 pounds much easier than I had imagined.

In fact, all I had to do was drive a few miles down the road and ask somebody for help.

Before

&

After

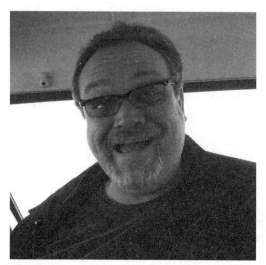

BEFORE: Scott at one of his heavier weights before beginning his breakthrough lifestyle transformation

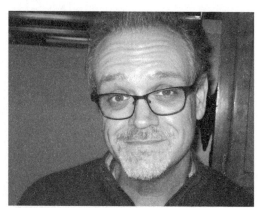

AFTER: Scott after descending to a healthier weight

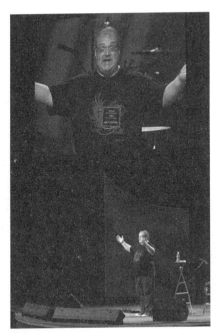

BEFORE: (Above) Scott is on stage and appears larger than life on the video screen behind him. **AFTER:** (Right) Scott performs at one of his concert.

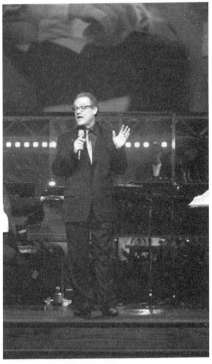

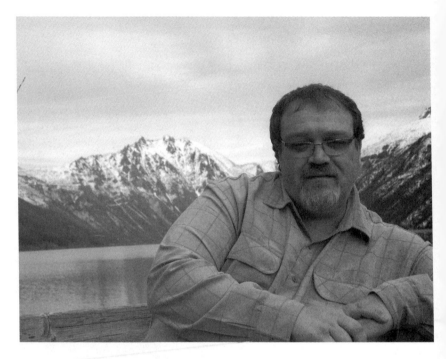

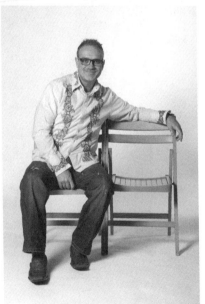

BEFORE: (Above) Scott pauses for a suave pose. **AFTER:** (Left) Scott shows how much less room he now occupies.

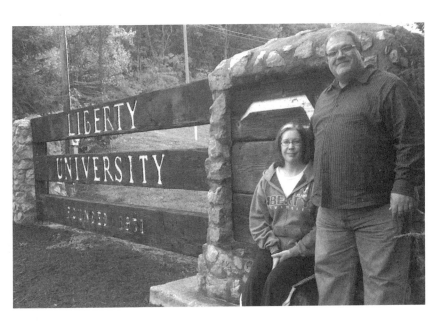

BEFORE: (Above) Scott poses with Donna outside the entrance of his alma mater just two weeks before embarking on his weight loss plan. **AFTER:** (Below) Scott points to Donna, who Scott gives a huge amount of credit for sticking with the plan.

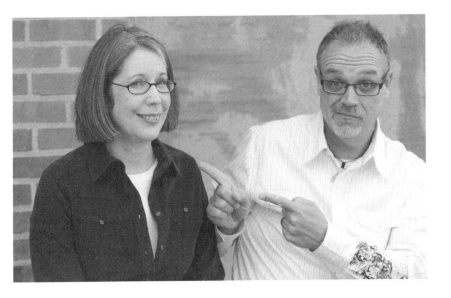

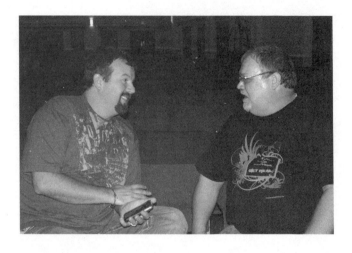

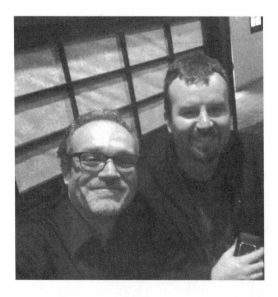

BEFORE: (Above) Scott talks with Casting Crowns' lead singer, Mark Hall. **AFTER:** (Left) Scott poses with Mark after trimming down.

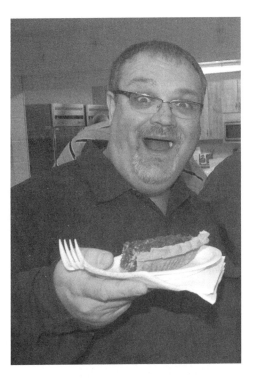

BEFORE: (Left) Scott can't help himself when it comes to pecan pie.
AFTER: (Below) Scott still manages to visit one of his favorite haunts, the Waffle House, but eats healthier there.

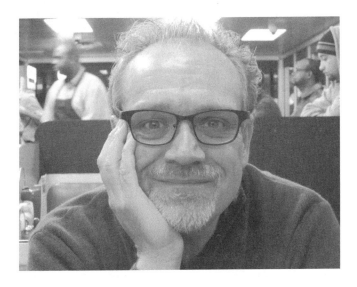

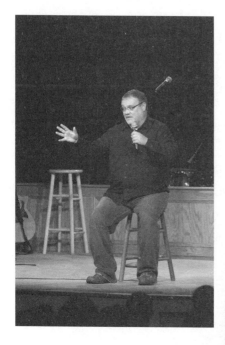

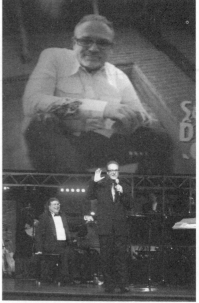

BEFORE: (Above) Scott takes a seat during one of his performances.
AFTER: (Right) Scott's jokes aren't overshadowed by his weight any more.

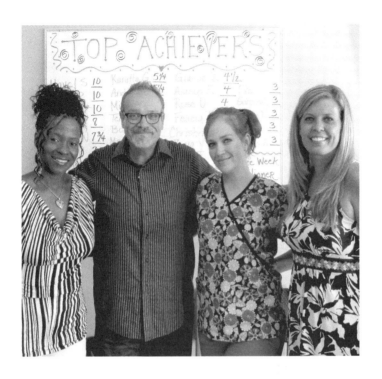

IN PROGRESS: (Top) Scott poses with the QWLCA team that assisted him, which included (from left) Diann Roberts, Scott, Amanda Littlefield, and Tina Couch. (At right) Scott's name appears at the top of the Southlake QWLCA leaderboard for most weight lost in a week.

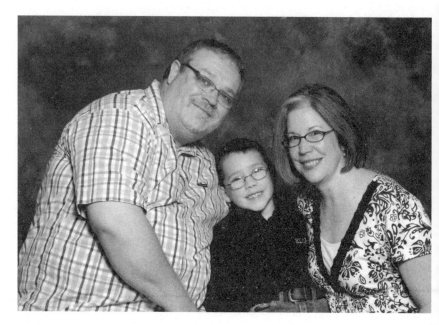

BEFORE: Scott and Donna pose with their grandson when Scott was near one of his heaviest weights.

AFTER: One year later, Scott and Donna posed with their grandson again after Scott dedicated himself to his weight loss plan.

Chapter 6

THE PLAN

"Supersize it—with a Diet Coke"

I sat at the restaurant table, reveling in the story my new waistline allowed me to tell. It's easier to smile ear to ear when your cheeks don't get in the way. "The diet includes more proteins than carbs, but it's not a no-carb diet," I said to my friend. I'll call him Mike. "They don't count calories, which in a strange way was freeing for me. I didn't feel like I had to toe such an exact line because I had freedom to choose among many options."

Mike grunted and nodded. Pass the pepper.

"They work with you individually, but basically you have two daily servings of proteins, four daily servings of vegetables, three daily fruits, and two daily starches, including breads. Certain foods on the list, like beef, you can have two days during a week but never two days in a row."

Mike bit into a megaburger, juices dribbling onto his chin. He didn't have room to talk, so I kept going. I noticed a guy in the next booth staring at me.

"They guarantee you three to five pounds of weight loss a week, and it's all in how you follow their formula, man or woman. It's how all the chemicals in the foods work together to create optimum weight loss," I said. "For example, there are a lot of great vegetables I'm allowed to eat, but certain ones I can't eat. They don't allow you to have peas because although it's a vegetable it's higher in carbohydrates, and other options are better. They want you to eat lower-carb vegetables like broccoli, asparagus, celery, cucumbers, string beans, and squash. I could eat, like, twenty-two different vegetables."

"What about fruit?" Mike asked, apparently in the pangs of guilt as he dipped another fry in his ketchup pile. The stout man in the next booth craned his head even more.

"The plan has more than a dozen fruits," I said. "I like fruit, and I'm allowed to eat stuff like grapes, blueberries, pineapples, and strawberries. I absolutely love strawberries. They make me want to cheat on the plan. But I can't eat bananas because they have more natural sugars that will slow weight loss. Same for pears—and for carrots in the vegetable category. And I can't eat any fruit after 6 p.m. But I get to chow down on grapes, apples, oranges, and grapefruit during the day. As a matter of fact, they use grapefruit as a 'breaker.' When you hit a wall and your weight loss slows, the clinic alters your diet with a breaker to help you begin to burn calories again. For me, they threw in grapefruit as a breaker because it speeds up metabolism."

Mike stopped chewing and looked up at the stout guy from next booth. He now stood at our table.

"Hi. I couldn't help but overhear you talking about your diet," the man said.

"Well, I prefer to call it an eating plan because it's really a lifestyle plan more than a diet," I said. "When I think diet, I think short-term or stop-gap."

"You're telling me," he said. He was rather large. "Gary," he said, sticking out his hand. Five minutes later, Gary had shifted his weight three or four times while standing beside our table before my courtesy kicked in.

"Pull up a chair," I said, and with that I added another hour on my restaurant stay. Gary wanted to know everything about my huge weight loss with QWLCA.

Mike finished his burger and licked his fingers. "You've talked about fruits and vegetables, but you haven't said much about the main course. Where's the beef? I bet meat is where they get you, ain't it?"

I resisted the urge to smack Mr. Carnivore with a smart-aleck reply. "Actually, just about the only thing I couldn't have is pork."

"You're kidding."

Gary widened his eyes too.

"I'm serious. I think I counted something like 42 meats on my plan. Beef, veal, poultry—I can eat chicken every day if I want—liver, fish, I can eat them all. I remember when they handed me my booklet at the clinic. I looked at the food list and thought, 'No wonder everyone raves about this.' The first section on the list includes ground sirloin, three different kinds of roast, and five different kinds of steaks, including sirloin and T-bone."

Gary's mouth opened slightly as he shook his head. Mike looked down at his plate apparently to make sure it was empty. I think I saw a faint frown.

For a little more than an hour, I outlined my metamorphosis thanks to the QWLCA plan. They peppered me with questions and leaned in to hear how 132 pounds melted off a 5-foot-9 guy whose sweatiest moment came under stage lights rather than on a treadmill.

This same conversation has repeated itself many times in different places over the past few years. Everybody asks, "How did you do it?" I've had total strangers walk up more than once to interrupt my conversation and say, "I heard you talking about your weight loss." They ended up pulling a chair up as I repeated details I love sharing.

The questions are always similar, and they reveal how entrenched Americans are in awful eating habits. The conversation usually starts with my long description of the foods and portions I'm allowed, and then come the questions:

"Well, can I eat pizza on this diet?"

"No," I say, and then tell them a few more items included in the plan.

"Well, what about ice cream? Can I eat ice cream?"

"No," I say, and keep going.

"Can I have spaghetti?"

"Uh, no," I say. "This is quick weight loss, not yearly weight loss. *Quick* weight loss."

It's funny how people's brains work. As I go into detail and say, "Here's what you do," I always hear the word "but," as in, "But can I eat this?"

> You have to be faithful and disciplined if you want to get healthy.

That's why many people can't lose weight. Their problem is their but. I want to say, "You keep saying 'but,' and that's what's going to keep your butt huge." Spoken like someone who used to need two trips to haul butt. In my old days, when someone would ask me "What's shakin'?" I'd say, "All four cheeks and a couple of chins."

My wife's mother is in her 70s. Donna told her about the diet, and even she asked, "But can I have this? But can I have that?"

No, no, and no. You have to be faithful and disciplined if you want to get healthy.

Don't look at what you can't have. Look at what you *can* have. Don't worry about the pizza. Instead, look at the plan and say, "Man, I can have steak twice a week."

It's been fun trying new things too. The QWLCA plan includes foods I never used to eat. I discovered veal is awesome. Dolphin? I've never tried dolphin. I think I'll try that soon. Lobster is on the plan.

Lobster? Are you kidding me?

The list includes sole. I didn't know what sole was until this plan. I thought it was in my shoe. Turns out sole is a flatfish like those in the flounder family.

The key is to dwell on the positive aspects. After a while, I found myself eating more variety than I did when I was fat because back then I ate only burgers and burritos.

Fast foods are basically the same junk from store to store, and it all kind of tastes the same.

Enjoying a variety of healthy foods is so much better than when I loaded up on a sackful of burgers and thought, "Man, this is going to be good." But I never felt satisfied afterward, and in a tape that looped over and over, I thought, "That really wasn't worth it."

If I ever start feeling sorry for myself that I no longer can eat pasta or pork, I try to remember the many nights of my burger discontent. I remember the consequences. It's the same as with sin: If we look past the fleeting pleasure to the consequences, we have a different view. It's never worth it because it's going to destroy us. The bad food just isn't worth it. It's unfulfilling, makes us feel bad, and ultimately will destroy us.

This fourth Golden Nugget is in the middle of my seven stages for a reason: It is the heart of it all. If you want to stay fat or get even fatter, make sure your eating habits include the same ol' routine of sticking your head out of the car window to yell into a drive-thru microphone: *Supersize It—with a Large Diet Coke, Please!* That Diet Coke is going to make all the difference in the world, you know.

At least it soothes the pesky Guilt Monster.

If you want to get as big as I did, you have to invent a meal between breakfast and brunch. You should never waste energy or time cooking or preparing anything. Make sure others in restaurants or fast-food joints do all the work for you. Commit unwavering trust into their capable, grease-coated hands.

Unfortunately, that routine supersized me.

The alternative is to develop healthy eating habits, and QWLCA offers the most effective approach I've tried. They taught me how to eat well and they loved me all the way through it.

Different

I want to stress the point that I didn't see this as a diet. I saw this as a revival, a manufacturer's recall, a return to what God designed. I simply broke bad habits, practiced good ones, and watched my waistline shrink. When it feels like your lungs have room to expand to draw more air, you know something is working.

This wasn't just a different lifestyle. This was a different life.

Two Old Testament verses describe my old way of life. Just as the Old Testament represents the old covenant of law, my old ways enslaved me to a system bound for death.

In two different books, King Solomon writes words I relate to my eating habits. Proverbs 18:7 states, "A fool's mouth is his destruction, and his lips are the snare of his soul." Perhaps Solomon meant to refer only to speech that mirrored the content of the heart. However, God convicted me to apply this truth to my old eating habits. My mouth served as a destroyer because those terrible habits overflowed from my heart as well.

In Ecclesiastes 5:6, Solomon writes, "Do not let your mouth cause your flesh to sin." My mouth caused me to sin multiple times daily, and my flesh had the stretch marks to prove it.

In my fat days, I microwaved canned foods or ate something right out of the can or box. I nuked giant Hungry Man meals and pined for more. I routinely downed two or three of them at one sitting. Donna and I opened cans of tuna and watched Food Network and said, "Oooh, wouldn't that dish be fun to try one day?" And then we took another bite of canned tuna.

Now we grill out, cook on the stove top, and chop our vegetables just like Bobby Flay. We buy squash, zucchini, and cucumbers, dump them into steamer bags, throw in a little Mrs. Dash seasoning, and steam them in the microwave. Two or three minutes later, out comes a delicious and healthy serving of vegetables.

Before QWLCA, I considered eating healthy time-consuming and costly. After all, marketers brainwash us into buying into the convenience and economy of "fast" food. Those are more of the devil's lies.

As you can tell by the descriptions of what I ate, I needed a second mortgage to maintain my old habits. Eating healthy is much cheaper if for no other reason than half the cows in New England are safe now.

Second, making a trip to a restaurant will never be faster than staying at home to grill and prepare fresh vegetables.

I'll challenge you to a contest. I'll cook one of the meals from my QWLCA book, even weighing my meat portions, measuring out everything, and firing up the grill, while you leave my living room to fetch a Big Mac. By the time you walk back in the door and kick off your shoes, I'll be watching TV and won't even be belching anymore. You would go to a lot more trouble, eat a much less healthy meal, and waste a few bucks of gasoline.

I always assumed cooking at home took longer because of the work required. If we're honest with ourselves, the reason most of us got big in the first place is because we prefer the easy road. For me, it wasn't that it took too long to prepare the food. It's just that I didn't *want* to prepare the food. I wanted someone else to do it for me.

God has set in place several universal, immutable rules. If I throw a ball off of a cliff, it's going down, not up. If I try to breathe underwater, I'll drown. If I tell my wife how to drive, at some point I'll get slapped. These truths are crystal clear to me. I had to learn the hard way that no shortcuts exist when it comes to health.

> I swallowed everything in sight, including the hook, line, and sinker of the myth that cooking healthy food is too hard, too tedious, too time-consuming.

I swallowed everything in sight, including the hook, line, and sinker of the myth that cooking healthy food is too hard, too tedious, too time-consuming. I crave immediacy, one reason I love to make people laugh. It's instant feedback. However, I learned it's not hard to chop up and steam a few vegetables, weigh and grill a slice of meat, and throw together a salad. My eating plan allowed one cup of squash during a meal. That's one squash. How long does it take to chop one squash?

Grilling is a breeze and doesn't require much cleanup, and Donna and I turned it into great bonding time. We were able to talk, watch TV together, or even entertain while we prepared and cooked our food.

This is how easy we made it: We love big salads, so we bought packaged, pre-washed mixed greens or spinach, threw in several nuggets of chicken from a refrigerated supply grilled en masse a few days earlier, dumped it all into a bowl, poured some dressing on top, and went to town. Without going to town.

How long does that take? Two minutes? In the old days, I hadn't even squeezed under the driver's wheel to go to Wendy's within two minutes.

When we eat healthy, time is our friend in more ways than one. It takes almost as long to microwave a frozen fast-food meal as it does to prepare healthy food. The good news is that while our nation has grown fatter because we supersized everything for years, the tide is turning. More companies, stores, and people are placing an emphasis on healthy alternatives. Supermarkets now carry entire sections of organic and whole foods. I couldn't say that only a decade ago.

Our Daily Bread

A typical day on the QWLCA plan requires three meals and two snacks. Notice I said the meals are required. The clinic insists on a routine to maintain the metabolism needed for weight loss. I couldn't skip meals, but I didn't mind. It meant I got to eat five times a day, which I needed because the plan's portions are much smaller than those to which I grew accustomed.

Out of respect to the proprietary aspects of the QWLCA approach, I will share one of my typical days to give you an idea of what is required and allowed. However, the only way you will lose weight like I did is if you follow QWLCA's two-pronged approach. The eating plan is important, but so are the visits to the clinic. Going solo won't work. Even if I copied the QWLCA plan verbatim in this book, you still would need to make the visits or phone calls and do everything the QWLCA way to forge lasting life change.

For breakfast at 8 a.m., I eat a piece of 40-calorie wheat toast with a fried or scrambled egg. I put the egg on the toast for a half-sandwich. I'm allowed one tablespoon of lite butter daily, and I use half of it on the toast before adding the egg.

I finish breakfast with one of my four servings of fruit. My favorites are grapes, apples, apricots, blueberries, cantaloupe, cherries, grapefruit, lemons, and oranges. For breakfast, I usually eat an apple.

That's not bad for breakfast. For a lot of people, it's a big meal.

At 10 o'clock, I enjoy my first snack. This is where I'm creative. At first,

QWLCA allowed me eight ounces of skim milk each day. After the weight loss, I can have ten ounces. For my mid-morning snack, I use the milk with another of my allowed fruits, strawberries, and a protein powder I purchase from QWLCA. I throw that stuff in the blender with some ice and whirr it around for several seconds. It makes a huge smoothie that holds me until lunch. Talk about yummy. I have to fight the urge to make more than one a day.

Poultry and fish are staples of the diet. Because the plan allows little salt, Mrs. Dash is my friend. Mrs. Dash is a line of salt-free seasonings that transforms a bland, flavorless piece of meat into a delight. I love spicy foods, the hotter the better. When I grill chicken, I alternate among different kinds of Mrs. Dash for variety. I love the Chipotle and Southwestern flavors.

It helps to eat foods with hot seasonings like cayenne peppers, raising metabolism to speed weight loss.

At lunch, I enjoy either an eight-ounce grilled chicken breast or seven-ounce turkey breast. I grill the chicken breast with a lot of Mrs. Dash and pepper. Mrs. Dash makes a marinade, and Donna coats the chicken with Mrs. Dash and sears it on medium-high. She adds no-salt chicken bullion cubes, turns down the burner to a low heat and mixes the bullion with water so the chicken sits halfway in the seasoned water. It simmers for an hour to ninety minutes. All the spices from the bullion cubes and Mrs. Dash combine to create a masterpiece of health. It is tender and can be chopped for salads or eaten in one serving as the daily eight-ounce chicken allowance.

The latter combined with two vegetables makes a fine meal. I can pick from asparagus, bean sprouts, broccoli, cauliflower, celery, cucumbers, egg plant, lettuce, mushrooms, mustard greens, okra, spinach, squash, tomatoes, and zucchini, among others. I also can eat kale, but I don't eat things that remind me of the weeds I spray in my lawn.

A neat bonus to the QWLCA plan is the cooking demonstrations during office visits. They often have a table featuring items they bought at a local supermarket. I learned about bullion cubes, dressings, and different kinds of butters—all of these wonderful goodies—just by watching the demos.

I keep my mid-afternoon snack quick and simple. My custom is to eat one protein bar. It has 15 grams of protein and somewhere between 170 to 190 calories, depending upon the brand. I buy boxes of protein bars from Wal-Mart or Kroger Supermarket because their brands are cheaper than the ones available at the QWLCA office yet have similar ingredients.

I eat dinner anywhere from 5 p.m. to 6 p.m., sometimes even later if I'm on the road. Standard fare is chicken or fish. Twice a week, I can eat a 5-1/2-ounce serving of one of the eleven choices of beef, but I can never eat beef two days in a row. It's that chemical thing again. I'm allowed two more vegetables for dinner, bringing the daily total to four servings.

The plan features great fish choices. I like to sprinkle Mrs. Dash on grouper or tilapia and place it on a ceramic plate at 350 degrees for twenty-five minutes until it reaches a beautiful golden brown. I steam veggies in the microwave, save my allowance of bread to make toast, and assemble a meal that should satisfy anyone.

The QWLCA people are ticky about mixing servings. For instance, I'm supposed to eat two vegetables at lunch and two at dinner. I cannot eat one vegetable at lunch and save three for dinner or skip vegetables at lunch so I can have an all-veggie dinner.

My two servings of vegetables often comprise a salad of lettuce and cucumbers. Sometimes I throw in the chicken Donna cooked in the bullion broth, and I prefer to use the QWLCA salad dressings because they are pre-measured for one salad. I don't have to think about it. I rip open the pouch, pour it on the salad, and dig in without worrying if I used the right amount.

Finally, I eat two servings of various starches each day. The selections include 40-calorie diet bread, melba toast, a bread stick, rice cakes, and Akmak crackers. That name scared me until I Googled it and discovered it's a healthy flatbread from a reputable bakery that's been around for more than a century.

Three times a week, I can have either one-half of a small baked potato or a helping of brown rice.

One of my weak spots is beverages—on this or any plan.

The QWLCA plan calls for mostly water, so it's wise to drink ice water with meals. I also can enjoy a daily total of two cups of either tea or coffee each day.

Honestly, I lost three to five pounds a week with no problem, just as QWLCA promised, but I didn't always follow the tea and coffee limitations. Sometimes I didn't drink just four or five cups of coffee a day. I drank four or five pots. Donna served as a nurse on the graveyard shift for years and grew accustomed to coffee. We have the large Bunn coffee maker that makes a pot in three minutes because we're coffeeholics.

It speaks volumes of the QWLCA plan that I ignored the rules and sucked down java like the caffeinated maniac I am and still shed the pounds. Maybe I tee-teed the pounds away. Maybe I jittered them off, I don't know. I guess coffee for me is like cigarettes for a recovering drug addict. I've got to have something in my hand, in my mouth, something to feed a compulsion—hopefully, maybe, one step at a time—until all the compulsions are gone.

I'm sure the plan still worked despite all the coffee because I diluted it. I had to drink eight to ten eight-ounce servings of water every day. Eighty ounces of water proved my biggest challenge. That's a lot of water. That's a lot of trips to the bathroom. I didn't know I could lose weight through my kidneys, but I did.

The water performed wonders for the weight loss and flushed out toxins while I burned off the fat.

A friendly suggestion: Don't drink all that water before a long flight. I learned that lesson the hard way. At least I had my customary aisle seat.

Here's a limitation I found interesting: QWLCA will allow you to drink diet colas but they must be clear sodas—like diet Sprite and diet 7-Up—because a certain chemical in colored colas makes you hungry. The daily plan permits two twelve-ounce cans of clear diet colas in addition to all other beverages.

I can drink all the herb tea I want, and I buy the brand offered by QWLCA. I call it poop tea. It's a natural laxative. If I feel a little backed up, I drink that stuff and the next morning the day begins great and flows naturally from there.

I'm confident you can find something you like on the QWLCA list of foods. If you're creative, the plan booklet contains recipes and you can mix foods and supplements and develop wonderful meals.

Consider these hints as "cheats," like the cheats in a video game. If I get really hungry before bedtime, I treat myself to a ten-calorie diet jello cup. Sometimes I add an extra vegetable of two cups of raw cauliflower right out of the bag as a snack. It gives me something to gnaw on and tames the beast.

Because the plan avails multiple choices from all food groups, I don't have to eat the same thing every day—here a cabbage, there a cabbage, everywhere a cabbage cabbage—and it helps break the monotony inherent in many diets.

I said I didn't have to eat the same thing every day. But here's the kicker: A lot of times I do.

I like routine. I found what I liked on the plan and for a lot of meals I stuck with it during the huge weight loss. Call it superstition. Or maybe my old one-track, addictive mind took over on some days. But when I saw the pounds evaporate like never before I thought to myself, "If it ain't broke, don't fix it."

No, spaghetti isn't allowed. So don't ask, even if the question comes with a but.

Small Bites

America's eating habits often are a double whammy. Not only do we eat unhealthy foods but we eat them in unhealthy portions. Sometimes I think the latter is most damaging. It's one thing to eat a slice of pizza every now and then. It's another to realize what you've done as you pick the last remnants of melted cheese from the bottom of an empty delivery box. Sometimes I didn't bother to remove the trace of cardboard paper stuck to the cheese.

The QWLCA plan limits portion sizes, an essential restriction for overeaters like me. When it comes to weight loss, the words *quick* and *second helpings* don't go together.

My plan's booklet lists specific portion sizes for every food. I can eat eight-ounce servings of chicken or seven-ounce turkey breasts. Most beef is apportioned at 5-1/2 ounces, most fish at either seven or eight ounces. I'm careful to purchase the correct amounts or weigh them pre-cooked. The majority of vegetables are one-cup servings, and I can have small to medium amounts of fruits.

If those amounts seem small it's because they are. I discovered I couldn't lose weight on the enough-to-feed-a-horse menu.

The QWLCA portions are closer to proper nutritional amounts than the servings I heaped upon my plate most of my life. The QWLCA plan retrained me to eat the way I'm supposed to eat.

While the QWLCA clinic publishes a general plan for everybody, it also adds customized steps for each client. Donna needed to lose less weight than I did, so she had fewer restrictions. At the bottom of the cover of my booklet, a staffer handwrote the following specialized instructions for me:

64 to 80 ounces of water per day
One-quarter to one-half teaspoon of Morton's Lite Salt
One tablespoon of Land O' Lakes Lite Butter
Two nutritional supplements
Eight ounces skim milk

While QWLCA makes available a line of helpful products, including not only vitamins and supplements but also salad dressings and protein powders and bars, they don't hawk them to you as soon as you walk in the door. Their supplements and vitamins are beneficial, but you don't have to purchase them. I didn't always use their brand.

Conservative radio host Rush Limbaugh used a supplement while on a Quick Weight Loss Diet in Florida. He lost 90 pounds and gave an unsolicited endorsement of the plan during his show. The various Quick Weight Loss Centers around the country didn't expect it, and their phones lines jammed over the next several hours. At least one Quick Weight Loss Center website saw so much traffic that two servers shut down.

I remember walking into the QWLCA clinic that day. The ladies scurried to pack vitamins and supplements and protein bars into shipping boxes. They told me it was because of Limbaugh's announcement. I didn't hear his endorsement, but I wonder if he talked about the easiest and hardest parts of the plan.

The easiest part is the exercise. The QWLCA people insisted I do none. Sold now?

I don't know all the scientific nuts and bolts of QWLCA plan, but they explained that all of these foods and portions work together to maximize metabolism. When I talked with Ron Presley, president of QWLCA, he discouraged exercise while on the plan, especially when you're larger. It apparently interferes with the process and can inhibit weight loss.

I know it sounds hard to believe. If you disagree, don't shoot the messenger. I'm just relaying the info and standing before the world 132 pounds lighter without working out.

First of all, I couldn't exercise. I couldn't bend over, much less run or climb on a Stairmaster. I could hardly put on shoes. I first had to lose a certain amount of weight just to be able to function.

I remember hearing of one lady at the clinic. She became upset when she had lost only half of her goal of forty pounds. They checked into her routine and discovered her rigorous exercise regimen. They told her to stop working out so she could reach her goal.

However, once you lose the weight, it's wise to begin exercising to maintain your weight and become physically fit.

After I lost the mass, my wife reminded me that loose skin looks no better than fat rolls when you're naked.

"So now let's get it toned up," she said.

But during the diet, the no-exercise rule is the easy part. Now for the hard part. One little handwritten line prompted a huge challenge: *One-quarter to one-half teaspoon of Morton's Lite Salt.*

Per day.

Ouch.

I slowly got used to it because I had to. It's the only way to lose substantial weight as quickly as I did. But I didn't like getting used to it. I had no idea I also suffered from salt addiction until this diet. It's amazing how much sodium we consume daily, and I learned how dependent on salt I had become. One-half of a teaspoon of salt is a tiny fraction of my previous daily intake, and the fact that it's Lite Salt added another degree of difficulty.

Such a limitation requires bearing down with unusual discipline. I weathered the storm and no longer enjoy foods seasoned with salt in amounts most people would consider normal.

You will notice my instructions stipulated one-quarter to one-half teaspoon of Lite Salt. That meant I had to have at least one-quarter teaspoon every day. They want you to have some salt (the chemicals!) but not too much because sodium causes water retention.

A requirement of any healthy eating plan is to stay away from processed foods. Most include salt as a preservative. In my fat days, I bought packaged sliced turkey and tore into it because I considered it healthy. I didn't realize I might as well have gnawed a salt lick like a cow. The sodium is excessive in most deli meats, canned sauces, canned soups, and even cereals. When Donna and I launched into the QWLCA program, we gave away every canned or packaged food in our home. That's another reason I love this approach—you don't eat out of a box. You get in a shopping routine and eat fresh foods.

Someone once gave me this tip: When you go to the supermarket, shop on the perimeter of the store. Most of the foods in the middle aisles are packaged. Everything near the walls is fresh produce, fresh meat, fresh fish, or fresh dairy. I guess it's cheaper to run electrical wiring there for the coolers.

Also, get into the habit of reading labels. It takes a little longer to shop this way, but at Costco I found frozen tilapia with no sodium and I can eat those large filets every day if I want.

Eating Out

One of the main questions I'm asked about this plan has a direct bearing on sodium intake.

"Can I eat out?"

The answer is yes. But it comes with a warning label: Sometimes you have to get rude. I'm joking, but sometimes it's as if the wait staff and cooks don't hear so good.

A terrific venue is Outback Steakhouse. They offer a steak that weighs about six ounces, meaning you leave a bite on your plate to stay at the 5-1/2-ounce limit. That falls in the Best Practices category anyway. The QWLCA strategy encourages ignoring what your parents raised you to do and leave a little food on your plate. Once you develop the habit of not cleaning your plate, it saves several pounds of weight gain each year.

At Outback or any other restaurant, I tell them to grill it plain, without butter, salt, or seasonings. I have learned to be specific because many times I had to return dishes to the kitchen. If it arrives drenched in butter, it has to go. I've almost cried before as the waiter turned to take the dish back to the kitchen.

"Can I just lick it first?" I asked.

The waiter laughed but realized I was kidding. I held my ground and developed better habits because the old Scott would've said, "Oh, OK. I'll just let it pass," and dive in. But that would mean breaking the plan, and the key to this plan is not to cheat.

A key factor to eating out is assertiveness. When I'm not direct and clear in my requests, sometimes the wait staff doesn't take me seriously. I make sure they know it's not a suggestion.

I remember telling some waiters, "Don't put any salt on it unless you want to see me keel over on the floor and die."

Their eyes got big as I looked over my nose and nodded my head. They scurried to the kitchen with their urgent piece of news. My wife laughed when

I did that because she's a nurse and knows we need salt to live. The waiter doesn't have to know that little tidbit though.

We regularly eat at many of the common chains (not fast food joints but cook-to-order restaurants), and we are able to find a dish within the requirements of our plan at just about any restaurant. We often place special cooking orders but have little trouble maintaining our diet. Sometimes we simply order salads with no cheese to make it easy on ourselves.

During my big weight loss, we ate at home more often since our old routine plopped us in restaurants almost every day. We still ate out while on the QWLCA plan, and the wait staff became our fans. We saw the same good folks over and over during the months of my weight loss, and they watched our progress and cheered us on. Even at Waffle House, we'd walk in and they'd say, "Oh, look at you this week."

Yes, Waffle House.

A lot of people ask me how I can possibly eat healthy at Waffle House. Nowadays, you can eat healthy pretty much anywhere. Even at McDonald's you can order a salad with no cheese. At Waffle House I order the grilled chicken salad. I replace the carrots with onions. Waffle House chicken breasts are bagged in their secret marinade. It tastes so good it must be laced with some kind of drug.

I told the Waffle House cook about my diet, and he surprised me.

"We can wash the chicken for you before we cook it," he said. "We do that for a few customers."

"Great," I said, halfway thrilled and halfway sad because the loss of the marinade. I knew it was too salty.

Every time I go to Waffle House the air is thick with those wonderful waffles. I feel like I'm sinning just being in the place. I always ask them to wash the chicken breast, and I watch them wash it right there in the sink and throw it on the grill. They chop it for the salad, and I bring my own QWLCA dressing. While Waffle House's own Lite Italian dressing has only twenty-five calories per pouch, it has a lot of salt.

I asked the QWLCA staff, "What do I do at all these restaurants that load their food with salt? I travel a lot."

"Buy a bottle of apple cider vinegar, and if you take a tablespoon at night it helps flush the salt out."

Almost every night, I take a swig of potent apple cider vinegar. I figure since apples are on the approved list, surely apple cider vinegar is OK. Strong as it is, even apple cider vinegar isn't enough to keep us on the straight and narrow when it comes to significant weight loss and life change. When temptation comes, we need help.

As I demonstrate in the next few chapters, I found all the help I needed in a good God, a good help mate, a good staff, and a good amount of willpower fueled by the momentum only significant results can generate.

Chapter 7

UP CLOSE AND PERSONAL
"Fly Solo, Where Even the Airplane Food Tastes Good"

On any given night at around two in the morning, flip over to QVC and you may hear the baritone voice of Scott from Stockbridge: "Yes, Julie, I love this broach. It's gorgeous."

When I finally married in my mid-30s, I needed two-and-a-half years to get out of debt from the junk I bought off of TV and stuffed into my closet.

Like the Gut Buster. Yeah, that really worked.

And then the Ab Lounge. My pastor says any exercise equipment with the word lounge in it ought to tell you something. I laid it in front of the fireplace to take naps on it.

I bought a treadmill from the Home Shopping Network. I used it for a week. Now I position my recliner beside it so I can kick back and watch TV while I walk my dog on it. I have a little leash to keep him safe, and he pants and drips and pants and drips and cuts his eyes at me and would cuss me in dog language if he had the breath.

I bought that little cow telephone. It's shaped like a cow, has spots like a cow, and even rings like a cow. Moooooooo.... Moooooooo. It's so annoying I can't wait for the answering machine to pick up. I won't even tell you what it does when I put it on hold, but it puts the chip in microchip.

I bought a voice-activated remote control for my TV. Have you seen one of those things? I scream into it: "Channel Five!" and it goes straight to Channel Five. It has a glitch though, especially when the TV is too loud. The nightly news teaser will come on and say, "Tonight at 11..." and, poof, it changes to Channel Eleven.

I'm enamored with the latest and greatest. Even if I don't buy it, I'm interested, and I love keeping up with the latest products. This fascination with all things new explains why I had to have the best gadgets during my weight loss. If I could figure out a way for something to help me lose weight, I wanted it.

I had a blender I used every day to make my strawberries-and-protein supplement shake. It was a good blender, but I always wanted the Vita-Mix brand blender, what I considered the Cadillac, Mac-Daddy blender. My juicer made too big a mess and I was too lazy to clean it up. Problem was, the Vita-Mix blender was expensive, like, the-wife-will-pout-for-a-week expensive. I never wanted to spend that much on a blender, and from the start Donna protested.

When I was single, I made the same amount of money as I do now but I had nothing to show for it except junk. I had every computer and electronic gizmo out there. When I got married, Donna put a stop to that. She's the boss when it comes to money, and for good reason. Sometimes it's like I'm a little kid and I have to work on her for a while. It took a year for me to wear her down and get that big blender. She said, "That's stinkin' expensive for a stinkin' blender."

I wore her down through a masterfully crafted guilt trip.

Honey, don't you want me to have every resource possible to be successful on my eating plan? This blender will help me eat healthy and lose weight. Don't you think it will pay huge dividends? What price tag can you put on my health? ....

I join several guys at my church to start each new year with a time of fasting and prayer. We've done this for four years now and it's grown from six guys to about fifteen. We pray and share weaknesses, trials, and struggles, and I cherish the time. I bought the original juicer to prepare for that week. I decided to abstain from solid foods but juice veggies to maintain electrolytes and nutrients.

I dreaded cleaning up after juicing, and my research sold me on the Vita-Mix blender. I can throw in whole vegetables and fruits, peels and all, and it liquefies everything. No mess. I bought it so I could drink everything without the cleanup.

I use it every day to juice vegetables and make soups. Back when Donna balked at the price tag, I tried to burn up the old juicer. But it just wouldn't die. I threw in all manner of stuff in bulk. She was in the next room and heard the blender struggling to grind: Whirrruuuuuugggggrrrrrrrrrrruuuuuuugggg. Then came tell-tale smell of an electrical burn.

Donna yelled at me. "You're purposely trying to burn that up so you can get the new one!"

"No I'm not," I said, waving my hand above the blender. "Whoooee, where's that smoke coming from? Hope the alarm doesn't go off."

My fascination with technology turned out to be a boon during my weight loss. I'm a fan of all Mac products. I have Mac computers for my marketing and promotions company, Third Heaven Imaging, and I adore my iPhone, iPod, and iPad. I keep waiting for them to come out with an iPizza because it would look terrific, taste great, arrive at your door on time, and be lighter than anything on the market.

Using my iPhone and iPad, I downloaded a couple of apps to chronicle everything I eat. This came in handy during my QWLCA checkups.

My favorite app is called *My Net Diary*. You enter your profile of how much you weigh, how much you want to weigh, and your exercise amount, whether it's sedentary all the way up to extreme. The app then calculates how many calories you should consume that day.

On the QWLCA plan, you don't count calories during the weight loss phase. Instead, you watch portion sizes and kinds of foods. You do the same during maintenance after you've reached your goal. It's helpful to count calories during maintenance since many more foods are allowed, and at that point the staff likes to keep track and assist you.

After I lost weight and reached the maintenance stage, I saw a health expert on the news. He claimed if you eat 1,000 to 1,200 calories a day, you will lose weight regardless of the food you eat. If it's cake, you'll still lose weight as long as you don't take in more than 1,200 calories per day. I can't say I wasn't tempted to try it.

His main point: If you eat the right foods, you can eat a lot and it would be a very healthy 1,200 calories per day. It's a misconception that 1,200 calories is not enough food. It just needs to be the right mix of the right foods.

When I go to QWLCA, I'm able to tap the *My Net Diary* app and hand the staff my iPad with a detailed list of everything I've eaten during breakfast, lunch, dinner, and snacks for a week. At the end of each day, it calculates the food I've eaten and provides my totals for calories, carbs, protein, cholesterol, and my Aunt Bessie's blood pressure reading. The detail is astounding.

I can type in my weight loss plan including my starting weight, current weight, goal weight, and target date to reach my goal weight. It then calculates whether I'm overweight for my schedule, provides my basal metabolic rate and body mass index, and prescribes the number of calories to consume that day if I want to maintain or lose weight. The basal metabolic rate is the amount of energy our bodies need to function at rest. This accounts for up to seventy percent of calories burned each day and includes the fuel needed for our hearts to beat and lungs to breathe.

The app also features an exercise chart to keep track of how many calories I burn in an intense workout or a morning stroll. It tracks water intake. It provides charts to help track weight loss. It has a library with tons of articles. It's a wonderful tool to keep track of your entire effort.

Another app called *Tap and Track* is a quick reference tool if all you want to do is watch calories. You can tap it and search the database for a burger and it'll show you its caloric value.

> If we eat too fast, we pack in so much food within twenty minutes that we're way ahead of the signal. By the time the signal hits, we're bloated like the Kool-Aid man.

I'm not getting paid to endorse any of this stuff, but I love the little apps. They help me even during the act of eating. I'm a fast eater. Though I lost weight, I still wolf down food. I go T-Rex on my plate and come up for air to see Donna finish buttering her toast.

That's a no-no. I've learned in the science of digestion our bodies need about twenty minutes to send the satiety signal to our brains. The communication says, "Hey, I'm full now. I don't need anything else."

If we eat too fast, we pack in so much food within twenty minutes that we're way ahead of the signal. By the time the signal hits, we're bloated like the Kool-Aid man.

With my iPhone, I'm able to tap an app and key in my information between bites. It helps me slow down. I'm not trying to ignore Donna, but it gives me something to do as I learn about the food on my fork.

At the beginning of my QWLCA maintenance, I chose to listen to the expert on the news and limit myself to 1,200 calories per day. It was my choice, and QWLCA didn't have anything to do with it. I examined what I ate on an average day and discovered that's about how much I consumed during my weight loss.

"I'm losing weight on that many calories," I said to myself. "So I'll try to keep it at that."

I got plenty to eat at that rate if it was the right kinds of foods. Donna couldn't eat it all on some days. She pushed her plate away several times.

I saw her leave leftovers one time and thought about another news report I saw on *20/20*. It featured a guy who eats less than 1,000 calories a day. He tries to consume no more than 700 calories a day and has been doing it for nearly two decades in an effort to push the limits of longevity.

The same report showed a caloric study with apes. One ape consumed 500 to 600 calories per day. The other ape ate whatever he wanted. The ape that ate fewer calories appeared twenty years younger than Sloppy Boy, who looked like I did after running through the airport.

The whole theory focused on the fact that we eat way too much in America, far more than God designed for us to consume. We're literally eating ourselves to death. The guy who eats about 700 calories a day is only 150 pounds and wants to live until he's 120 years old. With my luck, I'd be weak and delirious and step out in front of a bus at age forty-eight.

Some people would say, "I don't want to live that long if I can't eat. I'd rather die at 60 and be able to eat what I want." Yeah, well, I'd rather stick around for my family.

Based on all these latest news reports, it appears we've been duped into believing the daily caloric requirement is 2,000 calories. That's the figure the government and food industry consider an average for Americans, and it's the standard used on nutrition labels. You know how good the government is with numbers. Most people eat more than that even though many experts believe we should consume *fewer* than 2,000 calories per day.

After all, it's possible to eat 2,000 calories a day and grow to the size of Jabba the Hut on *Star Wars*. Two thousand bad calories are killers. The kinds of calories we eat can be just as important as the amount.

Try the Calorie Dare of eating 2,000 *healthy* calories in a day. Some people may not be able to reach the 2,000-calorie mark. It's a lot of food if it's the right food.

If we eat healthy, it's easier to stay under that threshold. A healthy salad of greens has few calories. A tasty piece of grilled chicken can have fewer than 200 calories. Asparagus and other veggies rate low on the caloric meter. Eat such foods three times a day and that's a lot of food and few calories.

Verbal Slap

Perhaps the biggest secret of weight loss is momentum. I'm not sure anything is more crucial than compounding interest. This term has more than one meaning for me. I needed something to hold my interest.

I have to see results to motivate me to continue. When I hear slow burn, I don't think of the safe weight loss rate of some diet. No, a slow burn describes how mad I get when my snail-pace diet won't let me have a slice of Mello Mushroom's jerk chicken and pineapple pizza.

I want to see and feel myself shrinking so my confidence goes the other direction. This is a huge reason for my fifth Golden Nugget: *Fly Solo, Where Even the Airplane Food Tastes Good*. If you want to stay fat or get even fatter, go it alone. Live and eat in a vacuum, where no one holds you accountable or challenges your selection of Ho Hos for supper.

In this area, the term helping doesn't refer to portion size.

I stayed faithful and disciplined on the QWLCA approach because it not only taught me an easy, low-maintenance plan for eating healthy foods but also provided the ultimate customer support. The QWLCA strategy includes real people who coach, encourage, and correct clients with amazing clarity and gentleness. And why wouldn't they? Most of the staff members were clients too.

I missed only a few days despite my busy travel schedule. I didn't mind the visits. The people were nice. Everyone in the office had used the plan to lose weight. They made it fun.

On Wednesdays, they provided motivation classes and cooked sample recipes. The group time built camaraderie. Before long, it felt the same as hanging out with a great small group at church. I wanted to keep my appointments because the staff had become friends.

They maintain a progress board on the wall. If you lose three pounds or more a week, you make the board. I saw where some people had lost as much as seventeen pounds in a week. I lost twelve pounds my first week because I was huge. It was mostly water weight. I think I tinkled it off, but I didn't care how it came off as long as it came off.

The progress board stoked me to keep going every week. When you see one of your advisers write a double-digit number on the board, it makes you that much more determined to match it or beat it the following week. It's like the home version of *The Biggest Loser*. It becomes a competition against yourself, the kind that is productive as opposed to Skinny Scotty vs. Supersize Scotty.

One week they weighed me and walked over to the board and placed my name in the top slot. I had lost more weight than anyone that week. I grabbed my phone and took a photo of the board.

The QWLCA staff kept things light. I didn't have to do what they said, obviously. And sometimes I didn't. Sometimes I walked in after eating an extra bowl of strawberries. Maybe two extra bowls.

"Oh, you can't do that. C'mon now," the ladies would say, and I'd take my verbal slap on the wrist and try to do better the next time.

The QWLCA folks asked me to record everything I ate each day to monitor my progress and make adjustments. I discovered it's a flexible approach. I also learned it's so finely tuned that eating prohibited foods or portions has an immediate effect. Even when I cheated by eating too many portions of an approved food, my weight loss slowed.

"Most people love our program, but we get a few people who complain," the QWLCA owner told me. "I get some letters from irate people who wanted to lose forty pounds and they only lost twenty."

He said his typical conversation went something like this:

Customer: "This is not working."

"What do you eat? Are you eating according to your plan?"

"Well, yeah, but I have to have my three glasses of wine at night."

"Then you're not following your plan. You're cheating. If you followed your plan, you'd still be losing."

He's right. When I plateaued after a while, QWLCA earned its money.

I had followed the plan almost perfectly and lost a lot of weight when my momentum bogged. They tweaked the regimen and introduced specific "breakers" to fan the metabolism flame. It reminded me of the times I worked out with weights and hit a wall and couldn't get past a 225-pound bench press. I had to do something different to push through the burn to get a new bench press max.

That's what QWLCA does. They change the diet and personalize it to find what works to crank the fat-burning dynamo again. I didn't eat cheese on the plan, but then out of the blue they allowed me to have mozzarella cheese for a few days. Don't ask me why or how, but it worked. It wasn't like I had strands of mozzarella hanging from the corners of my mouth, but I lost more weight the next week.

Sometimes the breaker included more protein and fewer carbs. I'm a meat-eater, so I didn't mind.

Once again, the accountability proved crucial.

I didn't have to think through this diet. I didn't count calories. They told me what to do and I did it. And when I stepped on the scales each week, the counterweights moved a little more to the left.

"Pick from these foods," they said. "Here's your proteins, here's your carbs, here's your vegetables, here's your fruits. You pick." So I did. Eight ounces of this. Three ounces of that. It was like ordering from a menu with terrific variety.

Most people who cheat on a diet will lie afterward. I've done that. On this plan, I learned to be honest no matter how painful the moment. The QWLCA staff and Donna reminded me to take ownership of my failures, my successes, my entire campaign.

Typical Visit

I lost 132 pounds in large part because of what I'm about to describe. Without my visits to the QWLCA clinic, without their policing and support, I don't lose the weight.

I believe the majority of overweight folks are like me—sometimes we need a pat on the back and sometimes we need a kick in the rear. My target was pretty hard to miss. I had to visit the clinic every business day for the first two weeks. If I didn't appear as scheduled—even during maintenance—they hunted me down on the phone.

A typical visit to the clinic started in my bedroom closet and chest of drawers.

I wore as few clothes as possible for an appointment that by necessity is up close and personal.

Every time you go in you're motivated and want to see you've lost weight, and clothes weigh something. It may be a few ounces, but that's a few ounces that ain't actually me. If you wear the same kinds of clothes and go to the clinic at roughly the same time every visit, your scale readings should be consistent. Your lightest readings typically come after you awake in the mornings and go to the bathroom.

I started showing up at QWLCA just before they opened. I stood out front in sweatpants, tapping on the door and fogging the glass as I peered in.

"Come on," I shouted through the door. "I'm going to start blowing up if you don't hurry."

I usually wore slip-on shoes. I've noticed young people sometimes wear pajama bottoms as their pants out in public. I was 47 but I wore pajama pants twice to the clinic. Donna scolded me. I just shrugged.

"Maybe people will think they're golf pants," I said.

I always carry keys in my pocket with two large chains full of keys. Sometimes I'm walking onstage at concerts when I remember to take off my key chains so I don't sound like the singing janitor clinking around. I always remembered to pull out my keys and wallet and take off my wedding band and watch before weighing. I even took off my glasses. Then I kicked off my shoes and climbed onto the scales.

One time I stopped at the clinic in nice clothes because I had another appointment afterward. I took a pair of sweatpants in a bag so I could change for my weigh-in. I wanted every advantage to stay motivated, and I knew sometimes clothes and shoes weigh four or five pounds. It takes a lot of cloth to cover a big boy. When I changed in the bathroom and walked out, the ladies smiled and shook their heads. I wasn't the first person to do that.

The QWLCA owner told me he walked in to the weighing area at one of his locations in Houston and stopped in his tracks when he saw a large lady standing buck naked in front of the scales, ready to weigh. Startled, he realized she refused to allow anything—literally anything—to get in the way of her weight loss.

I understood her desire. I wanted to see that scale drop every time, and I counted ounces. I weighed 201.2 ounces one time after weighing 201.7 the week before. If I didn't count ounces, then all I would've noticed is the scales stayed at 201. Instead, I benefited from five ounces of momentum. At the same time, it's discouraging to go in, step on the scales, and see no loss. And it's maddening when you've actually gained weight.

The key is never to give up.

That's where the counselors help. When you haven't lost weight or if you've regained a little, your tendency is to say, "Forget it. I'm headed to McDonald's. Then I'm going to go lay under the Frosty machine at Wendy's and have somebody open the spout."

The counselors step in and say, "It's OK. Let's change it up a little bit."

In one week they can help you escape a plateau.

After going in every day for the first few weeks, I tried to go in twice a week for the remainder of my campaign. I looked forward to the encouragement. You feel lighter when someone lifts you. Like meetings for Weight Watchers or Alcoholics Anonymous, you get the support of other people and make new friends and compatriots in a common struggle. We joked and laughed and had a good time.

I want to love people to Jesus, so I told them what I do for a living and talked about God and progressed toward sharing His story with them. Like Mark Hall says, "You have to earn the right to speak truth into people's lives."

> I looked forward to the encouragement. You feel lighter when someone lifts you.

After the weigh-in, the QWLCA staff took my blood pressure and recorded it. Then came the meat and potatoes, so to speak. Each session, a staff member took the time to sit down with me, review my food log (either handwritten or on my iPad) and counsel me.

They provide a booklet of general guidelines, but the most effective strategies came from my office sit-downs. They offered multiple approaches—Plans A, B, and C—and helped pinpoint the right one for each individual or for each week.

It's all personalized, and that's the reason it's important to make the office visits. I could hand you my QWLCA booklet and you might be able to pull off weight loss on your own. Yet the plan wouldn't be as intuitive or effective—and it certainly wouldn't be as fast and fun—as going to the clinic.

This essential accountability trains you to eat healthy and monitors all the little things that add up to big results. The staff ensures you get the proper amounts of water, salt, and fat content, like lite butters and oils. I could not have asked for better input. They even designed a travel strategy for me.

"I'm going to Seattle this week," I said, "And I'll have to eat in restaurants."

"All right, here is what you do. Make sure you tell the restaurants to cook it this way and do this and don't do that."

They even checked on me when I traveled. One day my phone rang while I was in another city, and I felt my jaw drop as I recognized the clinic number on my display.

"Is it going all right? Do you need anything?" the clinic worker asked. "Tell me what you ate, what you did."

And they'll slap you upside the head if you don't do it right—in love, of course.

After losing 132 pounds, I went on a maintenance routine in which I followed the habits I developed. But I added more variety (and occasionally cheated enough to regain a little weight; more on that later). Six months after I completed my big weight loss, they still called and loved on me.

Each visit takes fifteen or twenty minutes, depending upon how much I cut up with the crew. I never failed to get my money's worth, which brings up the next most pressing subject: cost.

Bottom Line

When I walked into the QWLCA clinic for the first time, I learned I could afford to lose weight in more ways than one.

I also knew by the end of the visit I couldn't afford not to do it.

The cost, like the plan, is different for everyone. You pay only for the amount of time you use the QWLCA clinic, and that time is based upon the goal weight you provide in your initial interview. They guarantee you'll lose a certain number of pounds per week if you don't cheat, and they're able to pinpoint the future week when you'll hit your goal weight. Then they charge you per week.

The less weight you have to lose, the less you have to pay since you pay based on the number of weeks you're in the program. It's not cheap but it's reasonable. However, the cost motivated me. I wanted to get what I paid for. It's human nature to do something half-heartedly when you have no real investment in it. I'm a firm believer in having skin in the game, especially when the skin needs liposuction.

If you hit a wall and need a breaker for a week, that doesn't count toward your bill. They help you get going again for free. They sometimes have promotional contests and announce, "If you lose more than three pounds this week, you get a free week added to your program."

The clinic asks you to pay the entire fee up front but will work out a payment plan if needed.

Inquiring minds always get around to the money. I love to keep people guessing on how much it cost me to lose all this weight and learn a new way of eating. Drum roll, please....

It cost me a little over $1,000 to lose 132 pounds. I paid about $7.58 for every pound I lost. That's the bargain of a lifetime—literally a longer lifetime. In the interest of full disclosure, I probably spent that much again on the QWLCA products, but that was my choice out of convenience. I didn't have to buy them.

What's the price tag on being around for Donna and my grandson when I'm sixty?

How much is it worth to be able to feel good about yourself?

I remember steamrolling through my weight loss, the pounds almost dripping off of me, and thinking, "If this cost $3,000, it'd be worth it for my health and other reasons."

People spend $3,000 for Lasik surgery to see without reading glasses. Losing weight can be infinitely more important than acquiring 20/20 vision. Either you do this and lose all the weight, or you hope no one else is getting Lasik surgery because you don't want them to see all your rolls.

The best endorsement I could give the program is that, knowing what I know now, I would do it all over again without hesitation. It was worth every trip, every minute, every dime.

And yet it was only part of the picture. I was so addicted to overeating that I needed more than just the QWLCA staff. I guess if Warren Buffet lived up to the way I prefer to pronounce his last name and needed to lose weight, he could afford to have the QWLCA folks go home with him. I couldn't.

I needed something else—someone else—for all the other hours of each day. In the next two chapters, I'll share how two friends made all the difference.

Chapter 8

SEVENTY-THREE CHIPS

"Dessert Your Will"

Carl Gates is my father-in-law. His mother and father died young. His brothers died young. But Carl is 76 years old and still at his high school weight.

He runs six miles every other day. He eats a healthy diet. Watching his disciplined lifestyle inspired me during my weight loss because my grand quest was all about mental discipline.

A disciplined person has a much greater chance of being a healthy person. In fact, my new eating regimen has helped me with my devotion time. If I can be disciplined in my toughest physical challenge, I also can be disciplined in my most important spiritual one (more on that later). I'm more disciplined to perform work for my ministries and marketing company. Not only am I more disciplined to do the work but I'm physically capable of lasting longer.

Inspiration fuels transformation. We all need motivators in various areas of life, but motivation makes all the difference in a pursuit as monumental as weight control. I know what it's like not only to be big but also blind and deaf. I had selective vision and hearing because I could tune out even the most inspirational videos, photos, and examples of people who had made themselves new in some way.

I don't know if it's accurate to say I tuned them out. I just couldn't hear them over my chewing.

Every year, Carl celebrates his birthday by matching his age with pushups. When he turned seventy-six, he did seventy-six pushups. He decided to battle the cycle of early death in his family by pursuing an active lifestyle.

Carl survived a motorcycle wreck a few years ago. Yes, he rode a motorcycle at age 74. I said he was physically fit. I didn't say he was bright.

He remembers riding his motorcycle one moment, and the next thing he knew he woke up in a Medevac helicopter. He suffered a punctured lung and several other injuries and needed months to recover but is at full capacity now. Doctors told him the mortality rate for his injuries to a person his age is ninety-five percent. For those who survive, ninety-nine percent wind up bedridden or in a wheelchair for the rest of their lives. It is obvious the Lord had His hand on Carl. Ultimately, God saved his life, but the doctors credited Carl's incredible physical conditioning for his full recovery.

And Carl owes his incredible physical conditioning to his equally incredible personal discipline.

Donna and I recently vacationed in Maggie Valley, North Carolina with her parents. One mile separated our hotels. Carl jogged to our hotel when he wanted to see Donna on Sunday morning. That's just Carl. When he runs an errand, he literally runs an errand.

I've always wanted to be that type person, but I learned a long time ago I can swallow good intentions right along with a slice of Red Velvet Cake. My fifth Golden Nugget addresses the ever-present temptations that haunt anyone who struggles with weight. If you want to stay mired in Tubbytown, then *Dessert Your Will.* Give in to those yummy, powder-sugared enticements that beckon at every break room, every vending machine, every company party. Gorge on the finger food even though it should be renamed fanny food since that's where it winds up. As a friend once said, "Eat, drink, and be merry... then die young and make a pretty corpse."

Most fat folks fall daily in this area. They simply can't say no to temptation.

Donna and I went on a recent shopping trip. While she slid clothes hangers across racks, glancing at the garments hanging beneath them—squeak (pause), squeak (pause), squeak (pause)—I sat in a corner and decided I'd stay productive. I whipped out my iPad, tapped my *YouVersion* Bible app and did a search on the word glutton.

Over and over again, I read the same pairing of words. In five of the seven verses that mention the word glutton, the words "drunkard" or "winebibber" also appear. For instance, Proverbs 23:21 states, "For the drunkard and the glutton will come to poverty, and drowsiness will clothe a man with rags."

That tells me something. Gluttony is like alcoholism. God puts them in the same category because of the correlation of the enslavements. I'm not sure if you're ever cured of being an alcoholic. I think you just have to stay away from it. It's the same for a glutton and his food.

Even in Jesus' day, people connected alcoholism with gluttony: "The Son of Man has come eating and drinking, and you say, 'Look, a glutton and a winebibber, a friend of tax collectors and sinners!'" (Luke 7:34).

As I listened to Donna squeak through the rack of clothes, oblivious to the truth bouncing around the chambers of my heart, the reality of how far I'd come dawned on me. I've never been liquored up, but if carbs and calories could pickle you, I'd be a dill by now. I can honestly say food intoxicated me.

Those of us who want lasting change must come to the conclusion that we are our own most formidable enemy in our struggle with self-control. We must endeavor to stand against temptation, knowing that God does not allow anything in our path, or on the caterer's table, that we don't have the ability to withstand.

While that verse gives us hope to stand against temptation, God also gave us common sense. It's a bit late to quote 1 Corinthians 10:13 while waiting for our change at Dunkin' Donuts.

If I'm an alcoholic, I do myself a big favor every day if I refuse to put myself in a position to stumble. If I have to go home a different way to avoid a temptation, it's worth it. Maybe the package store is on the easiest route home. Maybe every time I approach that store it seems as if a giant magnet pulls my car toward it. The wisest route is to go the long way home. It's the narrower road but it leads to life.

That means I don't go to Ryan's or Golden Corral or the Grand King China Buffet, where they have half of the Eastern seaboard laying out on hot lines. Every time I went to those places, I made sure I ate my money's worth. I wanted to make them wish I hadn't come.

Scattered, Smothered, and Covered

We all have our weak points. We all know exactly where we are most likely to stumble. Sometimes we stumble even when we brace for those moments. At other times, we breeze through the test, our resolve set because we guarded ourselves in anticipation of temptation.

Then come the surprises. Often, when we least expect it and just when we are feeling strong and self-assured, we walk around a corner and headlong into temptation.

The Bible says, "Let anyone who thinks he stands take heed lest he fall" (1 Corinthians 10:12). One of our most susceptible moments comes when we're riding high. The time right after a success requires an extra measure of caution. Human nature breeds overconfidence following grand moments, and right after I get full of myself I usually wind up full of crab meat.

It's tough to make a living on the road. Every church or venue I perform in, my host wants to take me to a nice restaurant. It's always a treat because I love to eat local specialties in hometown eateries.

People ask me why I love to eat so much. It's because I love the flavor of foods. I'm as addicted to zinging my taste buds as I am to filling my belly. While I was on the road, I never wanted to eat at the same old chain restaurants I frequent back home. We have Applebee's, Chili's, Longhorn, O'Charley's, just like almost every strip in the country. I want to go somewhere different in every city.

Artists who perform on tours often send requests for meals ahead of time. Because it is almost impossible to stay fit and disciplined amid the vagabond lifestyle, most artists ask for healthy platters or salads. In my bigger days, I sent requests for them to show me the best restaurant in town. I had one standard question.

"Which place has the best food that's not a fancy restaurant?"

Halfway through my concerts I sometimes thought to myself, "I need to hurry up and close. I'm hungry. Let's get to the closing prayer and go eat."

Food brought half the fun. I didn't mind if it was exotic as long as it was local. I'd eat any animal that didn't move or at least moved slowly. Buffalo ain't bad. Alligator indeed tastes a little like chicken, just more rubbery. And tripe is surprisingly good. Tripe, in case you don't know, is stomach tissue, usually from a cow. I've also eaten snake, emu, and squirrel. As long as it wasn't still twitching, I'd try it.

My curiosity led me to surprising discoveries at the oddest locales. The best barbecue I've ever put into my mouth was in Rapid City, South Dakota. I never figured I'd find some of the best Southern cooking in the country 70 miles from the Pine Ridge Indian Reservation. A couple from Memphis, Tennessee owns the little joint. My mouth waters thinking about it.

When I traveled with Mark Lowry years ago, we enjoyed looking for the best hole-in-the-wall restaurants. We called them Meat-and-Threes: our choice of meat for the day and three veggies.

My favorite always has been Southern food done well like my mother cooked. Lots of butter, lots of fried foods, lots of grease. Many people wouldn't be caught dead in a Waffle House, but I think I want to be buried in a casket that smells like the Waffle House.

It's easy to get fat when you awake at 3 a.m. and you're so hungry, so enslaved, that you're willing to drive to Waffle House and order hash browns that are scattered, smothered, covered, chunked, and topped. Southerners will know that means they're scattered and cooked well, smothered with onions, covered with cheese, chunked with tomato dices, and topped with chili. It's a thick pile of grease. And I hope it's on the menu in Heaven. I'd order the hash browns along with chopped steak and waddle home at 4:30 a.m.

Waffle House can be a world unto itself.

One night, I had the run of the place. I sat in the corner booth, listening to the unique conversation between the cook and two waitresses, the only other people awake in Stockbridge. The raging debate had many ins and outs, bold statements and subtleties. Points were made, others conceded. Heads nodded and shook, fingers wagged. And accusatory giggles filled the air. Their subject?

They argued about which county jail had the better food.

That's another reason never to cave in to late-night cravings. Mama always said nothing good ever happens after midnight.

On a different night I sat in my Waffle House booth and read a book. The waitress ambled up and said, "Whatcha doing?"

I looked up at her, then back down at my book and paused for a second. Then I looked back up at her.

"Reading," I said.

She looked puzzled and cocked her head. "What for?"

"So I don't have to work at Waffle House."

OK. I didn't say it, but I sure thought it. I didn't lose my witness. I was a fat Christian. But I was still a Christian. Besides, I needed her to bring me my favorite order.

Waffle House regulars will know this little recipe: I would order a slice of pecan pie and ask the cook to put it on the grill and dollop a big slab of butter on top. He put a steel cover over the pie and let the steam melt the butter into the pie. Oh, glory. It's indescribable. You can just hear your arteries hardening.

At other times, I took a piece of apple pie and had them put it on the grill with butter and then melt a slice of American cheese on top of it. How's that sound? I didn't think it'd be good until I tried it, and it's amazing.

I know this is supposed to be a book about losing weight. I know right now it sounds like a cookbook for tubb-a-lubs. Here's the point: All of this is Golden Nugget thinking. This is how to stay fat or get even fatter.

It starts in our minds. It starts with thinking about food, focusing on something we long for but don't have at arm's reach, and it creates desire even when we're not hungry.

Forgive the cruel method, but my reminiscing about my most terrible times of temptation played on your senses. You probably thought you were in a safe zone—a book about eating healthy and losing weight—and you were doing well. Yet the descriptions of my foraging at Waffle House carried away your mind to the all-too-familiar place of indulgence, and maybe my descriptions made you think of your favorite foods. Maybe you even smelled them. Maybe you're smelling them now....

Maybe I need to stop.

Temptation is a harsh minefield. It leads to sin, and I heard long ago sin will take you further than you ever wanted to go, keep you longer than you ever wanted to stay, and cost you more than you ever wanted to pay.

I so relished the taste of food and made it such a god that I would bow down and try anything. The food I described isn't something to desire. It's evidence of a crime. It's how I got fat.

Waffle House is a place I need to avoid (though I've found that I can eat healthily there if I remain disciplined). What's your Waffle House?

My Wife's Hand

Even dogs struggle with temptation.

I used to get my bowl of cereal, settle into my recliner, and prop up my feet on the coffee table to watch TV and eat. One day I finished this routine, took down my feet and put my bowl on the coffee table, then put my feet back up and continued to watch my show. Well, apparently the International Wife Manual says you're not supposed to do that.

"Huh-uh," Donna called out from the kitchen. "The milk will get all crusty on the bowl and the little bits of cereal will dry in the bowl and be too hard to wash out."

The whole time, my dog sat off to the side of the recliner, staring at the bowl. He made sure he was on the opposite side of the recliner from the tread-mill. He wouldn't get near the thing.

Every now and then, he looked over at me but then turned his head when my eyes met his gaze. Every time I looked at him, he turned his head away nonchalantly, acting as if no such bowl with no such trace of milk ex-isted.

It's as if he tried to say, "What? Me? That bowl? Pffft. Wouldn't think of it."

His little eyebrows twitched up and down whenever he'd look at the bowl or looked away. I finally broke down.

"Here," I said, and put the bowl on the floor.

He attacked it like it was full of filet mignon. Apparently that no-no is underlined in the International Wife Manual. I'm not sure which one hit my ear first, Donna's voice or the dishrag flying in from the kitchen.

"Scott! No!" she yelled.

"What?" I said, sounding like my dog. "He's been sitting there staring at the bowl. At least let him lick the thing."

I wilt under temptation even when my dog is the one tempted, but I stuck to the QWLCA plan religiously during my big weight loss. My visits at the QWLCA clinic helped. But so did the lady who threw the dishrag.

Donna truly was my better half during my great quest.

On the rare occasions I cheated while trying to lose weight, I cheated only with permitted foods. I might've had extra servings of strawberries or vegetables during the day, but they were on the approved list. I'm proud to say I never cheated on something off-diet like ice cream. I went for a whole year and didn't eat ice cream. I didn't eat pizza or pasta for a year. In fact, I haven't had pasta since November 2008.

I'm allowed to eat frozen strawberries. When I cheated, I ate maybe two or three servings of frozen strawberries instead of one because I love straw-berries. It slowed the weight loss a little bit, but on my initial surge of losing over 100 pounds I never had a weigh-in showing I had regained weight even when I slipped a little. I lost weight every week.

The QWLCA staff members reminded me they're human too. They all hear the call of the Brownie Siren like I do. The clinic offered me a new peanut butter protein bar during one visit, and the lady who worked with me said, "Oh, these are awesome. I ate a whole box of them one night."

I laughed because even the experts have those moments.

Donna doesn't. She's super strict. She's so precise in everything she does, even in her artwork for my company. I eyeball a piece and say, "That looks good to me." Not Donna. She blows it up to five thousand percent and counts the pixels. It has to be dead center. I tell her, "Nobody's going to know." She says, "Well, I know."

She's a little OCD about that stuff. I'm OCD about other things: I have to have exactly three steaks, cooked exactly medium rare. Donna's integrity helped me eat right every day during the campaign.

The QWLCA plan weaned me from pork. I occasionally dropped a few bacon bits on a salad, but those don't count because the crunchy ones in a bottle are Styrofoam sprayed with pork scent. Pork is forbidden because of high fat content. It's not like I can never eat pork again, but I have to moderate.

Understand, I love pig. My dad taught me I could eat every part of the pig, and I love the whole critter. Abstaining from pork has been tough because when I test on personality profiles it not only shows my gifts but also my passion for pork chops. During the maintenance stage after weight loss, the QWLCA plan doesn't include an absolute prohibition against eating certain kinds of foods. Rather, it encourages moderation and discipline. I wanted a lifestyle change rather than a diet because a lifestyle change has a greater chance of permanence than a diet. When you come off many diets and resume "regular" eating, you're going to gain.

Here, I must make a confession.

Donna asked me, "Are you going to be honest in the book and reveal you've struggled some in maintenance?" I looked at her and nodded like the sloppy puppy I am. "I think you ought to tell that, because that's where people are. They struggle with that."

I need to be honest. I regained about 25 pounds to reach 202 pounds after getting down to 177. But I reasserted myself as I pushed to finish this book, and I'm losing weight again. I plan to reach a new goal weight of 170 pounds, *less* than my college weight.

Now you know why I had success with the QWLCA plan in the first place. I can't overstate the importance of the regular visits to the clinic, but you can't take the clinic home with you. For someone like me, an unmitigated food addict, a plan partner is almost required. I'm convinced I could have lost weight alone because of my determination to change. Yet I know Donna's encouragement and correction, her mere presence, proved priceless.

It is imperative the people closest to us buy in to our weight loss efforts. Most people don't like conflict, and if the people around us don't support our efforts we would rather drop the effort than drop the pounds. It's just easier to pick up a fork than a dagger.

This is the sad reality for many overweight people. They want to lose weight and need help and support, but their loved ones poo-poo the need by refusing to sacrifice and eat right themselves. It's hell on earth to try to lose weight while a spouse is sucking down Haagen-Dazs.

Even the most stout-hearted warriors at the start of weight loss will fade without the love and support of family and friends.

Now, when I come to those lonely windows of the night that I used to call my Waffle House hours, I don't grab the car keys. I grab my wife's hand.

And I pray.

I thank God I have Donna, the personification of a biblical help mate. We've been married for 13 years and we're best friends. We laugh a lot and get along well, but when you get married in your mid-30s, you're kind of set in your ways. I want to do certain things certain ways, and she's the same.

We get along fine, but she still likes it when I'm on the road because that way I can't mess up her stuff or alter her routines. We've become my parents. When my dad retired, he drove my mom nuts because he stayed around the house all the time. He tackled projects like refinishing the cabinets and then put everything back in the wrong place. They fought more after he retired than they had when he worked and came home stressed. I still can hear mom saying, "Don't you have something to do?"

It's like that with Donna and me. We love each other, but all of a sudden she'll say, "Aren't you booked somewhere? When are you leaving again? I need some time alone."

In pursuing weight loss together we shopped together, cooked together, cleaned together, and read the plan together.

Donna lost 40 pounds on the plan and saw immediate results like I did. Two weeks into it, she began experiencing radical changes in her health. Her hot flashes and night sweats disappeared long before substantial weight did.

Here's why: I think everybody's strength is also his or her weakness. For instance, when it comes to my ministry, the people who work with me know

I'm particular and tough. It's got to be done right and on time even though I'm not personally organized. My hard edge sometimes gets on people's nerves because it sounds like I'm mean when I'm really not. I'm just demanding to make sure the performance is good.

In the same way, Donna lost weight because she is precise about doing things. When she starts something, she is completely devoted.

Her dad convinced her to start running one year. They found a race every weekend—3K and 5K runs. Friends joined Donna as she ran races all over the state.

When she started running, she wasn't quite up to shape but she finished the race no matter what. If she turned red and bordered on a heart attack, she still would cross that finish line.

"That's the way you were with this diet," I told her the other day. "Once you decided you were going to do this, that was it."

That helped me because I knew she was going to be strict at home, on the road, at the restaurant, or wherever.

At the same time, her strength is her weakness. When she went off the diet, if she was going to slip up and have a doughnut she was going to do it right. She was going to scarf a whole bunch of good donuts with ice cream on top.

Thankfully, those moments have been few and far between.

We've trained ourselves to eat healthy meals in healthy amounts, and our proven track record assures us we can continue it. The joint effort bonded us more closely than we've ever been, and not just because our bellies are no longer in the way.

"We shared a common goal," she said recently, and that is true. The same reasons motivated us both and we worked as a team. I'd prepare part of the meal in one half of the kitchen and she'd work in the other. I'd chop squash, and she'd work on the chicken. Even now, when I grill I go buy the chicken and she does the prep and seasoning. I grill it while she prepares the salads. Then we enjoy the fruits of our teamwork.

We usually don't sit at the table though. After coming off the road, I like to use TiVo to catch up on our favorite TV shows. But it's not like we're the Cleavers. We bicker, but I think it actually helps us eat right. She's not afraid to call me out or slap my hand. I'm thankful for her obsessive tendencies when it comes to my eating.

Donna read an article the other day that asserts couples that argue live longer.

"Well," I said. "We ought to live to be 150."

We're like best friends and laugh a lot, but we go Edith and Archie on each other all the time. I've learned if she's really mad about something to give her time and she'll get over it. And then she'll apologize to me because usually it's her fault.

Even while losing weight I sometimes tried to be sneaky. Remember, I'm the guy who hid wrappers in the trash and snuck out at night.

"No, no, no," Donna said more than once. "You already had your three fruits today. You can't have a bowl of strawberries."

"It's OK," I said. "I'll drink some more poop tea and get it out."

Donna rolled her eyes.

"Or I'll use prunes as one of my fruits," I said. "That way, if I eat it's going to come right back out in a few hours."

Donna sighed and shook her head. "You're an idiot," she said. "Some of your logic is just so weird."

I like Mexican food, but it's hard to eat healthy on Mexican food. It's possible, but the options are not so grande. After losing my big weight, we decided to test a local Mexican cantina. At the table, I whipped out my iPad.

"What are you doing?" Donna asked.

"I'm writing down stuff. I'm counting the tortilla chips we have."

"It doesn't matter if you count them. You still had seventy-three chips," Donna said. "Just because you're counting them doesn't mean they're not fattening."

I slumped my shoulders, looked at the ceiling, and filled my cheeks with air like a blowfish. So frustrating. Once again, she was right.

"Yeah, you're counting your calories, and you just had 4,372," she said. "Set your limits."

I'm thankful I have Donna to help me set them.

Good Advice

Someone asked me about my toughest, lowest moments of weight loss and whether in those moments I had thought about Christ's temptation in the desert.

After fasting forty days and nights, Satan approached Jesus with a proposition. The devil said, "Hey, if You're really God's Son, command these stones to become bread. Prove who You are. I mean, if You're God then You created the rocks in the first place and it's nothing for You to make bread out of them."

Satan taunted Christ and sought to lure Him out of God's will and to bow to his wishes. That's his age-old technique. He always has something better for us, something easier, something full of half-truths. Every single time, it caters to our flesh.

Jesus, exhausted and starving, didn't bite:

"It is written, 'Man shall not live by bread alone, but by every word that comes from the mouth of God'" (Matthew 4:4).

Jesus quoted Scripture, and He did it not just to defeat Satan at that moment but also to demonstrate for all of us how to combat the enemy. The Word of God is our most formidable weapon in this immensely spiritual and mental war, and Scripture has the power not only of spiritual salvation but also of physical victory. This truth begs the question: How can we use Scripture in our most desperate and pivotal moments if we don't know Scripture?

I like to find the most powerful Scriptures that relate to my struggle and commit them to memory. Throughout this book are several wonderful passages that can serve as useful answers to temptation and cravings. It is an exhibition in power beyond yourself to be able to stare at the sheet cake at the office party and say, "I will set nothing wicked before my eyes; I hate the work of those who fall away; It shall not cling to me" (Psalm 101:3).

The verse before that one is perfect for a placard in our dens: "I will behave wisely in a perfect way. Oh, when will You come to me? I will walk within my house with a perfect heart."

Knowing the truth is one thing. Appropriating it is something else. I can write all of this truth because I know it to be effective truth, but I didn't always invoke it. Yes, during my lowest moments I thought of Jesus' response to temptation. I also thought of the Krispy Kreme doughnut I wanted to stuff whole into my mouth.

I'm a practical guy as well as a spiritual guy. While I believe quoting Scripture is the most powerful spiritual *and* practical step we can take, I also use other strategies to help survive what I call those "temptatious times."

Eating habits either can be a defense against temptation or a cause of temptation. Good habits lead to a good defense. Bad habits generate temptations.

Donna and I went to Longhorn Steakhouse recently, and she ordered the chicken and asparagus. She ordered it right off the menu with no special cooking instructions like we asked for during our big push for weight loss. They brought out the chicken drenched in seasonings, the asparagus slathered in butter.

"I don't like this," she said. "You can't taste the asparagus because of all the butter and salt."

After that experience, Donna now orders the same meal but uses the special instructions because it tastes better. Her taste buds are renewed because her mind is renewed.

Before trying QWLCA, Donna and I would go to the movies and she'd get popcorn and dump in so much butter that the popcorn almost floated. Then she'd take the salt shaker and hold it high—I guess so she could see it—and it would rain salt on the popcorn. She'd shake it up and pour more salt. Shake it up and pour more salt. Then she'd wrap the salt shaker in a napkin and take it with her into the theater. She didn't steal the theater's shaker. She just borrowed it. She always put it back after the movie, but she wanted to salt the popcorn as she went through the bucket.

These days, she turns up her nose at salt. Why? Because salty food is only a habit. She ordered French Fries for the first time in a long time the other day. She took one bite and said, "Whoa, the salt on there is incredible."

In my fat days, I made my own trouble. Isn't it interesting how we'll sit down to watch TV and then get up and go stare into the refrigerator and think, "Oh, I have nothing to eat in this house"? Then we open the cabinets only to find slim pickings before moving on to the pantry. Finally we settle on something the roaches wouldn't eat and return to the TV. Thirty minutes later, what do we do? We go back to the same refrigerator and stare again as if the food fairy brought something new in the last half-hour.

The QWLCA plan teaches several good habits to combat such cyclical moments:

Set a routine. Establish meal and snack times and eat only during those times. Forbid yourself to eat anything else at any other time. And get ready to quote some of that Scripture. You'll need it.

Set an eating place. This is a subtle but helpful strategy. You wouldn't think eating in one place in your home could have much of an effect, but it does. Just ask your dog. Pick your spot at the table and eat only there, even for snacks. I need to work on this because I like to park in front of the TV. If you don't give yourself permission to eat anywhere else in the house, you'll train yourself to go to your spot and confine your "feeding" there. And don't get offended when your dog sounds like Smedley and laughs under his breath.

Pursue other interests. One of the most effective strategies in weight control is to avoid boredom by engaging in favorite activities. If those activities eventually include physical activity that burns calories, all the better. I avoided eating when I was hungry by reading my QWLCA plan booklet or working on the computer or reading the Bible or praying. Sometimes Donna and I went for walks, and now we like to bicycle. Hunger pangs go away when your mind is focused on something else.

Use smaller plates. Much of eating is psychological. I've seen normal people load up their plates only to get halfway finished and say, "My eyes were bigger than my stomach." I've never had that problem. I learned we can trick our brains into thinking average portions are larger than they really are by using smaller plates, even if you have to buy some. If you can't afford new plates, spread out average portions on your plate (rather than piling them) to achieve the same effect. Your mind sees less plate and believes you're eating more than you are. This technique convinces the brain to be satisfied with less.

Disobey your parents. If your parents were like mine, they taught you to clean your plate. This discipline likely stemmed from the Great Depression and also from the days of more rural living in our country. It became almost sacrilege to throw out perfectly good food. If you want to lose weight, don't clean your plate. Leave a little out of principle.

Reward yourself. Divide your weight loss goal into achievable stages and reward yourself when you reach a marker. If you're trying to lose 100 pounds, then treat yourself to something you really like for every ten pounds you lose. You don't get a milkshake, but maybe you get another cool pair of shoes.

Don't leave leftovers. Prepare and cook only what you plan to eat. Leftovers are a chilled temptation when you stand and stare with the fridge door open.

Don't stand and stare with the fridge door open. There is no such thing as a food fairy. If you find yourself doing this, it's because you're bored and need something to do. Go back to Good Habit number three and pursue other interests.

Follow these guidelines and, at the end of another day of success, you can head off to bed content that you honored God by living up to yet another valuable Scripture—just like the psalmist who came through trials and temptations with unwavering faith.

"You have tested my heart; You have visited me in the night; you have tried me and have found nothing; I have purposed that my mouth shall not transgress" (Psalm 17:3).

Chapter 9

THE DEFINITION
OF FREEDOM

"Place Your Order Anywhere but at the Lord's Table"

M y monumental lifestyle change wasn't the first time I'd shed significant weight. Before Donna and I married in 1998, I got down to 195 pounds. I weighed well over 200 pounds for years but felt my biological clock ticking, which at my size was Big Ben. I knew I had to lose weight to find a woman.

I found her through her daughter, Brandy, who attended the student ministry I helped lead. Brandy knew I was a performer because her family had watched me in most of Mark Lowry's videos. She introduced me to her mother, and we took it from there, much to Brandy's chagrin. It meant her master plan backfired.

She had thought, "I'll introduce mama to this guy. He'll introduce her to Mark Lowry, and she'll marry Mark Lowry."

We know this to be true because years after our wedding Donna found a letter written by a teenaged Brandy to Mark Lowry. She wrote Mark all about her mother and how she'd make a great wife. Donna found it because Brandy never mailed it, and we discovered her motivation for introducing Donna to me.

Talk about tugging on the heartstrings of the second fiddle.

I was 36 when I got married. I thought I knew all about women. I now realize I knew nothing about women. I mean, I didn't know toilet paper had a certain way to roll until I got married. Just this past year, she convinced me it went on that little stick.

As a bachelor, I'd leave clothes everywhere. I like to get comfortable when I come home. When I hit the door in my single days, I'd leave a trail of clothes from my welcome mat to my recliner because I'd get comfortable on the spot. After we married, Donna grew flustered with my act.

"Why don't you pick up those socks?" she said.

"Honey, if you give 'em long enough, they'll go to the laundry room on their own." I knew I was in trouble when she didn't laugh.

I learned more about women when I took my dirty dishes to the dishwasher. I want a dishwasher that will live up to its name and actually clean a dish. Many fall short of their purpose. One night, Donna tried to train me on proper dishwasher use.

"You've got to prepare the dishes for the dishwasher," she said.

"What? Prepare them? It's a dishwasher."

She filled the sink with water, poured in dishwashing liquid, and grabbed the dishrag and sponge and Brillo pad and buffer and sander and drill and readied every dish for the dishwasher.

"That's like painting the house before hiring a painter," I said. "You just washed it before you wash it!"

I don't want a dishwasher like that. I want a dishwasher so strong you can insert a plate with a chicken leg stuck to it and when it comes out the chicken leg is gone. I want a dishwasher that will do what it's designed to do.

This is why I decided to try QWLCA. I also wanted an eating program that does what it's supposed to do.

An observation by Mark Lowry on my wedding day reminded me for years afterward that I needed more than just a typical diet. Mark served as best man at my wedding, though he tried to bail.

"I don't know if I should be your Best Man," he said. "Everyone I've ever been Best Man for got divorced."

Donna and I are still going strong, in large part because Mark obeyed Donna at our wedding. Donna told him he couldn't open his mouth until the reception, and he didn't cut up at all. But he said something that day, when I was 195 pounds, I'll never forget.

"I know you, Scott," he said, cutting his eyes at my slim waistline. "You're going to say 'I do' and head to the buffet."

Mark is a great funny man and singer but apparently he's also a prophet. I guess he knew our honeymoon was a cruise. Like Mark says, all you can do on a cruise without sinning is eat. Of course, the way I went about it was sin.

At first, I followed the disciplined regimen I planned. I promised myself, "I'm going to eat only sugar-free desserts on the ship." I planned ahead to order all the healthy options. Gyms on cruise ships are as big as the gym I attended back home. We booked a seven-day cruise, and I just knew I could maintain my discipline for a week, even a week outside my normal routine.

I ate my diet stuff for the first couple of days. I went to the gym and lifted weights, ran on the treadmill, and sat in the sauna. On the third day, I used only the sauna. On the fourth day, I watched other people work out. On the fifth day, I passed the gym on the way to the pizza buffet.

I wound up eating the midnight buffet. Just as Mark predicted, I started gaining weight on the cruise and did not stop for any extended period until I started the QWLCA plan.

The final and most important ingredient to the recipe of good health is the one most overlooked even by Christians. We need to take it to God. The ultimate diet partner, the ultimate helpmate, the ultimate encourager is the Lord. This is why the final Golden Nugget to staying fat is *Place Your Order Anywhere But at the Lord's Table*. Wide is the road that leads to approaching weight loss in your own strength. *Very* wide.

The only way to guarantee success on this plan or any other is to take everything to the Lord. A clinic full of experts helps. An encouraging loved one or friend is crucial. But it is possible to lose weight without those folks.

In my opinion, it's impossible to change without the Lord's help.

Focus

The Apostle Paul in his second letter to the church in Thessalonica encouraged believers to "pray without ceasing" (5:17). This means our days are to be filled with a constant conversation with our Creator, most of it under our breaths as we request wisdom and discernment, ask forgiveness, pray for others, and seek strength and boldness.

We must depend on Christ and His strength to maintain good habits and good health. He won't solve our problems for us, however. He doesn't hand life to us on a silver platter, especially when we're licking our chops to see what's on the platter. He promises never to leave nor forsake His children (Hebrews 13:5b) even when we continue in destructive habits. He stands patient, opening doors of escape and wooing and inviting, the loving Father awaiting the wayward child.

God won't do everything for us, but He will go through life with us and help us beyond measure. It's comforting to know Jesus is with His children through the tough times and good times. Mark told me something years ago I consider profound: "God not only loves us but He *likes* us."

I suspect the statement resonated with me because of my past. I grew up in an independent Baptist church, and we served God almost out of fear. I feared God would strike me dead in high school when I looked at a pretty girl the second time.

God wants the best for our lives. It's like the Christian teenager who wanted to go the party on Friday night. Everyone knew about it, and everyone planned to go. She came from a conservative, godly family and she wanted to go hang out with friends. Ultimately, she decided to stay home. Her friends asked her why.

"What, are you afraid you'll get caught and your dad will hurt you?"

"No," she said. "I'm afraid I'll hurt him."

We should live for God not out of fear He will hurt us but out of fear we will grieve Him. Our parents want to be proud of us. They want us to succeed. I'm motivated by my desire to please my heavenly Father and to refuse to do anything that will displease Him. That relieves the burden of the performance-based theology of my youth. Everything was how you looked, who your friends were, what you did, what you said, and where you went.

It's not about doing. It's about being. It's about who you are in Christ. It's not about dwelling on some back-and-forth battle between flesh and spirit. It's about abiding in Jesus and learning to enjoy Him. My problem during the incessant war between Skinny Scotty and Supersize Scotty was misguided focus. I had my eyes on my gut rather than my God.

A focus on the Lord brings strength and resolve. Only then can we walk past any buffet line, hear the dumpling demon whisper, and answer in full confidence of the Lord, "Sure, I'd love to dive in. But that's not me anymore. I'm not my own. Jesus owns me. Jesus is my life."

When Jesus walked the earth, most of His family thought He was nuts. They couldn't figure out the man who had grown up with them but now performed inexplicable miracles for perfect strangers and spoke in mysterious parables weighted with eternal truths. They couldn't wrap their minds around the fact that the kid who fetched water with them now walked on it. They knew Him only as a brother, not God's Son.

Then something happened.

After Christ's crucifixion, He arose from the dead and opened the way for anyone who would believe in Him to have eternal life. Because He lives, we can too.

That's exactly what happened to at least some of His family. First Corinthians 15:7 reveals that Jesus' half-brother, James, saw Jesus after the resurrection. James knew what had happened on the Cross. He knew Roman soldiers rolled a heavy stone into the doorway of Christ's tomb. He knew they sealed the stone over the entrance. He knew the soldiers stood guard over the tomb.

And James knew, sometime shortly after the Resurrection, Jesus stood before him with nail-scarred hands and feet. The Bible does not give details, but James' reaction must have been similar to that of Doubting Thomas. When he saw the resurrected Jesus for the first time, Thomas uttered one of the most powerful pronouncements ever recorded: "My Lord and my God."

No need to reach and touch the scars. Just....

"My Lord and my God."

In my heart, I believe James did the same. I believe this because James went on to become the pillar of the Christian church in Jerusalem, abandoning his forefathers' Judaistic faith that had convinced him Jesus was a lunatic. Before Jesus' crucifixion, James looked at his half-brother and scoffed because he knew better.

After seeing Jesus alive again, James *really* knew better.

I love how James begins the only book of the Bible credited to his authorship. He identifies himself in the first sentence: "James, a bondservant of God and of the Lord Jesus Christ."

Bondservant. That means slave. Before he was martyred for his faith in Jesus, James earned the nickname "Camel Knees." He prayed so often and for so long that his callused knees looked knobby like a camel's. Imagine the moment he gazed into the resurrected Christ's understanding eyes and everything changed.

Jude, another of Jesus' skeptical half-brothers, also has a New Testament book credited to him. Guess how he opens it?

"Jude, a bondservant of Jesus Christ and brother of James."

Bondservant.

The brother they once disowned they now bow before. The fringe lunatic they once mocked is now their forever Lord.

That, to me, is the definition of freedom. I want to be enslaved to Christ so I may be free of all the encumbrances of this world. Call it a crutch and call me weak, but I'll always call Him King.

I laughed when Mark Lowry said, "Hey, there are relatives I have to love because they're kin to me. That doesn't mean I want to go on vacation with them." But God not only loves us, He likes us. He wants to spend time with us. He's crazy about us. To me, just as a great friend wants us to be the best we can be and succeed, including in the area of weight control and all the inherent struggles, God wants us to succeed as well. We should lean on Him, seek Him, and trust Him.

But how? How do we trust Him with weight loss? What does it mean to take this to the Lord? It means:

We realize the real battle is spiritual. The key to victory over weight control is to recognize this isn't the battle of the bulge. It's a battle for the heart and mind. We are spiritual creatures—the real you is the spirit inside that oversized bag of bones—and therefore everything that touches our lives has spiritual implications. In Ecclesiastes, Solomon writes, "All the labor of man is for his mouth, and yet the soul is not satisfied" (6:7). He's saying what we stuff into our mouths can never bring lasting peace and contentment. Our struggle isn't physical, it's spiritual. It has psychological, emotional, and mental ramifications, but the battle is spiritual. Take care of the spiritual foundation first, and the rest has a way of falling into place (see Matthew 6:33).

We spend time in Bible study every day. This is how we take care of the spiritual foundation. Through study of His living Word, God renews our minds to rid us of old habitual thought patterns and retrains us to see ourselves and others as He sees us. Psalm 119:103 states, "How sweet are Your words to my taste, sweeter than honey to my mouth!" Now we're talking eternal dessert!

We pray. And then we pray some more. Why? Because there is power in prayer. We pray to start the day. We pray to close the night. We pray through the cravings. We pray for strength. We pray for courage. We pray for protection from temptation. We pray during temptation. We pray for discipline and consistency. We pray to sense God in every bite. "Oh, taste and see that the LORD is good! Blessed is the man who takes refuge in him!" (Psalm 34:8). Nothing rivals the flavor of the Savior.

We obey. When the Holy Spirit whispers in His still small voice that a particular menu item has too many calories or too much salt, we don't pretend we can't hear Him. That still small voice may as well be a megaphone at that moment, but sometimes we out-talk God. That's when we wind up burping lasagna. But it's not lasagna that sits on our stomachs two hours later. It's an extra helping of guilt.

We ignore the enemy's taunts. Yes, we have fallen. Yes, we feel the extra helping of guilt. But failing doesn't make us a failure. It makes us human. A key to weight loss is ignoring Satan's giggles and false accusations when we stumble. His lies are a mirage. They're like a Hollywood movie set, extravagant and convincing on the outside with nothing behind them. They feel heavy but weigh nothing compared to the gravity of God's truth. When God convicts, He convicts about a particular sin. He is precise because His Word is sharper than any two-edged sword. When Satan accuses, he generalizes. *You're a bad Christian. You're a loser. You're a fatty. You'll never get the weight off.* When we stumble, we ask for forgiveness if we have sinned, and we start again, same nose to the same grindstone. God's precious Word trains us how to recognize Satan's lies and believe truth instead. Then it's up to us to never give up. Ever.

Matthew 6:33 states: "But seek first the kingdom of God and His righteousness, and all these things shall be added to you." The "kingdom of God" refers to the rule and reign of Christ not only over the universe but also in our hearts. That's why Jesus said the kingdom of God has arrived. It's already here because He came and He reigns.

"All these things shall be added to you" means God takes care of the rest. When our focus and lives are centered upon Him, God has our backs. Thankfully, He's strong enough to have my front as well.

Taking everything to God means a daily offering of our lives—every fiber of our being—to Christ and submitting to His authority. We are to ask Him for strength and should trust Him to provide everything we need to persevere. This isn't a head game. It's a heart reality.

One verse later, Jesus gives us a final, crucial assurance: "Therefore do not worry about tomorrow, for tomorrow will worry about its own things. Sufficient for the day is its own trouble."

In other words, live the cliché: one day at a time. Don't worry about how tomorrow will be impacted if you mess up today and fall off the wagon and land in the buffet line.

Tomorrow is a new day. Start fresh.

Revival

I can think of no better way to close this final chapter than to share some of the benefits of my weight loss. The results are worth the trek. I have seen a revival in my spiritual, sexual, and physical lives.

When I think of the QWLCA plan, the first word that comes to mind is discipline. The second is intimacy. They may seem unconnected, but I found they are interdependent.

It's easy to assume losing weight spices up your sex life, but you have to live it to appreciate it. It's amazing what losing a spare tire does for the engine.

Donna and I are having more fun because we have fewer rolls to get past and it's not a chore anymore. Donna used to frown and say, "Oh, I've got to do this?"

I don't collapse into bed from fatigue anymore. Before, I climbed into bed and asked, "You wanna do it? Well, come over here because it's too much work to roll over there." It's like anything else. You have to have energy for it. Now that I'm slim I like to remind Donna that studies show sex burns calories just like walking and running. I smile and wiggle my eyebrows at her.

"We need to burn some calories, baby. It's part of the diet."

If a man and woman are married, God wants them to have intimate relations, and my intimacy with Donna is much better now that we've lost weight. Sometimes sex is involved, sometimes it's not. The improved intimacy includes times we lie in bed and talk. And we talk and talk some more. That intimacy has deepened. It correlates with the intimacy we want with God, the kind in which we can share anything with Him and go as deep as we're willing.

A life-changing challenge, even if it's one we didn't ask for, often has the result of drawing loved ones closer to each other. In our case, the weight loss also pulled us closer to the Lord. He empowered the weight loss to begin with, and we talked to Him more as He helped us persevere.

In the intimacy of prayer, we don't have to pray a King James prayer. We should talk to God like He's our best friend, because He is. He knows our struggles. He knows our weight problems, addictions, sexual issues, loneliness, or whatever we face. He wants us to kneel before Him, lay it at His feet, and be transparent—even when we need to complain.

Sometimes I have to vent to people just to get something off my chest. Donna sometimes says, "Why are you mad at me?"

I have to tell her, "I'm not mad. I'm just venting. I just need to get rid of it."

It's OK to vent to God sometimes. He'll listen. God is God. It's not like you're going to change His essence with your words. Yes, He is holy. He is all-powerful God. Respect Him? Of course. Honor Him? Of course. Worship Him? Of course—but worship Him in spirit and in *truth*.

Part of that truth is being willing to talk with Him about everything. He already knows everything anyhow. It's not like we ever surprise Him. Prayer is for us, not God. An unchanging God gave us access to Him for prayer to change us, not to change His mind. We should come to Him boldly, as the Bible instructs, and that means we should boldly be ourselves because He knows us anyway.

In another conversation, Mark told me, "Never ask questions of God accusatively, but it's OK to ask inquisitively." Instead of saying, "Why did you let this happen to me?" say instead, "Why is this happening to me, Lord? Teach me. This is hard. It's no fun. Nevertheless, not my will be done but Your will be done."

We are laid naked and bare before Him to whom we must give an account, the writer of Hebrews says. Goodness gracious, if He's going to see that hideous sight, why shouldn't we be blunt and honest with Him?

Marriage is a spiritual union, and my wife and I are closer spiritually after this monumental undertaking. We tackled a shared goal, achieved it, and learned mutual lessons along the way. It motivated me to think, "Hey, why can't we have a shared goal in Bible study or in prayer?"

When we discipline ourselves in eating and weight control, it correlates with how we react to God and how we practice the spiritual disciplines of Bible study and prayer. It correlates with the discipline of obedience, where we let our yes be yes and our no be no.

I've noticed undisciplined people often are undisciplined in most areas of their lives, including in matters of ethics. This discipline deficit often shows during perhaps the single most difficult hour of the week—when the alarm clock goes off on Sunday morning and launches the first salvo in the mental battle of rousing the family and heading to church.

We're supposed to forsake not the assembling of ourselves because God knows we need each other. Satan does too, and that's why he puts sleeping gas in the ceiling fan on Sundays.

Now that I'm healthier I'm awake more often to study my Bible. I'm trying to get back to studying Scripture in-depth. I read in short spurts. But when I was fat, my spurts still weren't short enough. I couldn't hold out. I stayed groggy, my brain a pickled haze from the flush of foods, and I'd conk in the middle of my study. I'm embarrassed to admit that on more than one occasion I got down on my knees to pray and the next thing I knew it was 6 a.m. I fell asleep on my knees by the bed.

I've fallen asleep while lying in bed and talking to my wife. As I drifted, I snapped myself out of it to make sure I paid attention, but then I'd hear a faint, "Scott, are you listening to me?" You hate to do that with your wife or with God, but at least God is more patient.

I'm more alert now. I don't fall asleep on either.

In my fat days, I often was asleep before the plane taxied to the runway and I didn't wake up until someone nudged me as people collected their bags from the overhead compartments to deplane. On my trips now, I may take a small nap but usually I'm wide awake. The first time I stayed awake I looked down and thought, "Oh, look. They have magazines in the back of the seats. I never noticed that."

Another spiritual benefit is I'm awake to share the Gospel with people on the plane. I haven't done that in years because of my size and drowsiness. I've been convicted about it because I've sat on the plane before and thought, "OK, if I don't say anything, maybe nobody will bother me."

Years ago, when I first started flying, I took advantage of witnessing opportunities with my captive audience. I've had people pray to receive Christ right there in the airplane seat. I am burdened to witness to people more often, and now that I don't drool on them anymore they're more receptive to the Gospel.

The New Me

I always heard the clichés that significant weight loss restores energy and stamina, and now I know it's true. I even have more time in the day. I go to bed earlier and rise earlier. I sleep less but I sleep better because I don't have sleep apnea. I'm not waking up wheezing, coughing, and gasping for breath.

I'm not getting up multiple times to go to the bathroom and verging on diabetes with dry mouth.

I walk places whenever I travel now. Before, I stayed in my hotel room. Donna and I went to Las Vegas not long ago. I did a concert at a church but stayed a couple of extra days for Donna to celebrate her birthday there. The city's slogan is, "What happens in Vegas stays in Vegas." She figured if she turned another year older while we were out there she could come back home and the extra year would remain in Vegas.

I did my concert on Sunday and spent the next three days enjoying one of the benefits of weight loss. I don't get as winded anymore.

We stayed at the MGM Grand, a great hotel. But, again, I'm cheap. I rented the cheapest room, something akin to a closet. In fact, housekeeping kept knocking on the door not to clean it but to ask for toilet paper and bottles of cleaner. They thought it was the custodial closet. It was tiny.

We planned to use the Internet at the hotel until I saw the fee. I don't know why big hotels charge you through the nose for Internet access. Go to Microtel or Motel 6 and you get free Internet. Go to a posh joint and you need to see a loan officer to surf the web.

We decided to walk to Starbucks for coffee and free Internet access. I didn't realize until I looked up directions on my iPhone that Starbucks was more than two miles away. We walked the strip for 2.2 miles. I never would've been able to make it when I was tubby. I would've paid the exorbitant Internet rate to keep from having to leave the hotel. It rejuvenated me to discover I wasn't winded when I reached the coffee shop.

I had a membership at Gold's Gym one year when I was big. I went four times all year. One day I lumbered over to the treadmill and cranked it up. I set the pace on Three, which would seem slow for most folks but felt pretty fast for a 300-pounder.

Now I average the same speed I tried on that treadmill but I do it for exercise while Donna and I talk, enjoy the fellowship, say hello to neighbors, and get to know people.

When you're too big, you lose out on many small pleasures. I'm actually able to bend over now. I can always tell when a big person ties his shoes because the shoestring knot is always off to one side. Crazy as it sounds, I have enjoyed a mental boost and motivation knowing my shoestring knot is in the middle again. Just wearing shoes with strings feels like a return to normalcy.

I didn't anticipate a shrinking waistline would make my house bigger but it did. I had to get rid of a ton of big clothes. I've been to Goodwill probably six times in a little over a year, and I'm still finding 3X and 4X pants and shirts I never plan to wear again.

My closet is probably two-thirds empty. I'm slowly buying new clothes, shopping for nicer items at more fashionable stores. Quality or designer clothes often are cut smaller. It's rare to find them for big and tall people. Instead of draping material over me that happens to be sewn together in a massive seam, I can wear form-fitting shirts from nicer stores. I'm still cheap enough to search out the clearance rack, but dressing nice makes me feel a little better about myself. It's a reward for my hard work. I'm more confident, and it shows even in my conversations.

Another benefit is I can sit on an airplane and not feel like I'll need a crowbar to get up when we touch down. Perhaps this little achievement isn't important for everyone, but when you travel to make a living, airplanes and airports are a way of life. I also have slack in the airplane seatbelt. Before, I was right on the verge of having to use a seat belt extension. I had to use it twice on smaller planes, but on the big jets I was barely able to squeak by without the humiliation of needing the extension. I've seen others do the Hand Raise of Shame to request the extension, and I thought, "I don't want to be that way." It made me mad at myself that I was even close to that point.

Eric Jackson, my road manager of eleven years, traveled with me during my behemoth days and watched me suck in my gut and pull the seatbelt so tight it appeared stretched thin in the middle when I buckled it. If it had snapped and hit a flight attendant in the forehead it would've killed her. I was a walking weapon of mass destruction and Mr. TSA never knew it.

But now, I punch Eric in the ribs and say, "Lookie there. Ain't that cool? There's two feet of slack." I laughed out loud the first time I did it.

Even walking down the airport concourse is different. In the past, Eric had to carry everything because I was worn out. He hasn't traveled with me as much lately, but I don't need him to carry my stuff anymore. I can do it now. I even walk up flights of stairs. In the past, you may as well have asked me to scale Everest. On my rare trips to the mall or anywhere else that has steps, I skip the elevator and use the stairs as exercise.

Donna's weight loss produced unexpected results. She's more alert and no longer has hot flashes and moodiness. Bless her heart, she can be moody.

(Have you ever noticed when a Southerner starts a sentence with "Bless her heart" something bad comes next?) Sometimes, she can be mean. One day, I called her Sybil and asked her which person was planning to show up that day. I found out which one real fast. Eating healthy changed the chemicals in her body, made her feel better, and improved her mood.

Which improved my mood.

As portly as I got, I never experienced depression. I guess I fit the mold of the quintessential fat, jolly guy. Donna has battled depression before, and I didn't understand it. When my wife dealt with clinical depression, nothing else was wrong with her except depression. Our marriage was fine. Our finances were fine. Her work was fine. We got along fine. Still, depression gripped her. I didn't know what to do. I've been down before, but I don't grasp depression because I've never been there.

I angered Donna when I'd say, "Just go out. Do something. Have fun. Go to the store. Shop. Let's just get out and go." She wanted to ring my neck. It was like a skinny person looking at me when I was 300 pounds and saying, "Just quit eating. Put the fork down. Chew." As if the notion had never crossed my mind.

When I was big I thought to myself a million times, "All I've got to do is not put food in my mouth. Just DON'T DO IT." But I'd do it anyway, moth to the flame. I had to remind myself of my eating woes when it came to Donna's depression. "I have no clue what's going on here," I finally admitted, "and I don't know how to handle this depression stuff. But I'm here for you."

We're both grateful her weight loss and healthy eating regimen balanced her body chemistry. She's in the maintenance program now, and when you're in maintenance you don't always follow the plan's strictest prescriptions. You can try other foods, sometimes just because you miss them. I can see attitudes change when we haven't eaten the right foods. I can see more irritability in both of us. This is when it dawned on me the food-to-chemistry matrix is as dynamic as the QWLCA folks claimed.

Time to Sweat

I have lauded the QWLCA plan for helping me losing 132 pounds without exercising. While it is true I was so overweight I could not exercise when I started the plan, I would be unwise not to take advantage of my new body through exercise.

I actually want to work out now.

Donna and I saved up and invested in two nice bicycles. Our grandson, Dylan, is seven now. His dad bought him a yard sale bicycle to use at our house. We decided to buy cruising bikes so we could go on rides with Dylan and also exercise when he's not visiting. We ride about every other day. Panola Mountain State Park is near our home, and the state of Georgia has paved about thirty miles of connected bike trails from Panola to Stonecrest Mall. Our goal is to be able to ride the entire distance.

Of course, Donna is as detailed as ever. She spent a month researching all things bicycling. At the bike store, she stared at the serious bicyclists clip-clopping around in their special riding shoes with the pedal clips.

"They ain't messing around," she said. "Do they have to wear those funny clothes—those Speedo-looking things?"

"I'd look good in that now," I said.

She snapped her head around. "Trust me. No, you won't."

Yep. Depression's gone. She's her old self again.

Instead of my reading coupons for Wendy's and Burger King, I pore over the new bike magazine and read all about cycling. Even my reading habits have changed from food to exercise. I'm getting into it and enjoying it, but having somebody along for the ride helps.

I looked in my closet and found the old Ab Lounge device I bought off of QVC. Now I use it for the purpose it was designed instead of taking naps on it. I have a 300-pound set of Olympic weights with a bench and rack along with pushup grips and a pullup bar, and I've started using my equipment again. I could hardly sit up at all a few years ago, and now I can exercise.

Mark Lowry can't tease me like he used to. He used to tell me I did one situp a day—half in the morning when I got out of bed and half at night when I went back to bed.

Life is different. I'm blessed to have another chance to take better care of what God gave me.

I look back at the long afternoons full of "errands" and all the clandestine late-night hamburger runs and want to weep at the wasted time and the sheer debauchery of it all. As easy as it seems to stigmatize people for the damage drug and alcohol addiction causes and the victims it creates, I've learned to be less judgmental. Their chemical dependence is simply a different formulation than mine. Granted, food isn't illegal and doesn't leave you drunk or high, but isn't it just as big a crime to allow food to incapacitate your life, your zeal, your effectiveness?

I'm on this planet for a reason, and I'm quite sure it has nothing to do with satisfying my gut. My soft underside brought hard lessons from a hard recovery, a kind of rehab I never envisioned I'd need.

I bow my head and thank my God, my Jesus, the One who makes all things new, for granting me a new beginning.

I hope He always reminds me of why He did this. It wasn't just so I could live longer. It wasn't just so I could feel better or even feel better about myself. It wasn't so I could write a book. It was because, as He said in the first beginning, I have a purpose wherever I go and in whatever I do. I'm supposed to enjoy a relationship with Him and to love Him, honor Him, and obey Him. I'm supposed to glorify Him. And now I can look in an unfogged mirror without hesitation and know something else He said in the first beginning.

I'm also supposed to look like Him.

> *"So God created human beings in his own image, in the image of God he created them. ... God saw all that he had made, and it was very good."*
>
> *— Genesis 1:27, 31*

May we always give Him reason to see Himself in us. May He always be able to look at us and say it is very good.

Conclusion

Lord, Have Mercy

I heard about a gentleman who smoked for decades before finally quitting. He said it took him five years of not smoking before he no longer had cravings for a cigarette. Five years. He didn't smoke during that entire five-year span, but he struggled with the pangs of wanting something in his hands or in his mouth, something with smoke to blow.

Donna says he should've hung around me for a while. I can blow smoke with the best of 'em.

But think about battling that urge for five years. I believe I face a similar challenge. It's going to take time to rid myself of the drive to eat whatever pops into my mind. I anticipate a long process. I know I'm still ascending the front range.

You hold one of my primary motivations for staying the course. I don't want to blow up again after writing a book. I told somebody I was writing a book about my weight loss and they shook their heads and smiled.

"Wait five years and then write a book if you're still thin."

I see the wisdom in that. But I welcome the pressure of staying true to my word. I'll use anything at my disposal never to go back. Once I say it I'd better live up to it, and it's going to be tough because I do love food. I love fattening food.

I've come full circle. I had to make up my mind to start this eating plan and new lifestyle, and now I have to make up my mind to stick with it. I'm convinced I'll remain in a healthy cycle if I continue to do the opposite of my time-tested Golden Nuggets.

I admit it's been difficult to maintain good eating habits. In fact, it may be harder to make up your mind to stick with it than to make up your mind to start it. I love food so much it's hard to ignore some foods forever.

My church recently had a cookout. Chef Darren Hughes presided. Darren is the sound technician for all of Casting Crowns' tours, but he's also a grillmaster. He grilled ribs, hamburgers, hotdogs, and turkey sausage. I skipped most of those without a second glance.

My problem came when he rolled out the Fried Oreos. He literally batters Oreo cookies and drops them in a deep fryer. I'm convinced they'll be on the banquet table in heaven. Lord have mercy, they're unreal.

Somebody had to stop me on the way back to my table. I had about four of them on a plate.

"No, no, no, no," my friend said. "Put those back."

"They're for Donna," I said, mostly serious. I wound up trying one. Later, that friend told Donna the Fried Oreo story.

"I know. He really struggles with food," she said. "He'll stop by Krispy Kreme and bring home a dozen doughnuts. I'll say, 'Why did you get the doughnuts?' He'll say, 'For you.' He loves to watch me eat. He enjoys it vicariously. That's his love language."

I guess I'll have to stay stuck in the last chapter of this book, constantly grabbing Fried Oreos and Krispy Kreme doughnuts and having to take them to the Lord.

It helps to hear the reactions of people who see my weight loss, however. I know I'm not supposed to base my sense of self-worth on what others think or say, but the truth is I get a boost when people notice the big difference in me.

I've actually had someone say, "Oh, you look good. You're the same guy?"

A young lady on my staff once worked as a church secretary. While she still worked at her church, I accompanied Billy Lord when he appeared as a guest singer there. We chatted with the young lady in a back room as we waited for Billy to go onstage.

The subject of my Get Real conferences came up. I conduct these conferences on evangelism and spiritual revival at Christian schools, and Billy helps me. The young lady recognized Billy from one of the conferences she had attended a few years earlier. I was quite large when the woman saw me onstage at the conference.

She raved about the conference to Billy. I sat there listening to her but she had no idea who I was. Billy said, "Well, you know, this is the guy who started the whole thing and does most of it."

"That's the guy?" She looked stunned because I don't look like the same man. That moment has happened several times in different contexts. It's a bit disconcerting—a mix of embarrassment, relief, good pride, and male ego awash in one.

One of the tellers at my bank couldn't get over my change.

"You've lost weight, haven't you? You look good." She went on and on about my appearance, and I said, "Well, thank you."

"No, you look really good. I mean, you look *good*." For a second, I thought she wanted to give me her number.

I guess that's better than the old days when I wouldn't have gotten hit on by a walrus in heat.

In my first few months on the QWLCA plan I lost forty pounds and not a soul noticed. I grew a little discouraged even in the middle of tremendous personal success. Guess whom I called? My buddy, Mark Lowry. I suppose I'm a glutton for food *and* punishment.

"Man, I'm frustrated," I said. "I've lost forty pounds and no one notices."

He went into that thick Southern drawl and said, "Keep it up until it shoooows."

After I lost all my weight, I talked to Mark again. I let him know I had kept it up until it shows. He congratulated me, of course, but Mark is Mark. He couldn't just leave it at that.

"Do you have skin hanging everywhere?" he said.

"No, it's drawing up."

"Good," he said. "People need to lose weight when they're twenty, not when they're older. Skin doesn't draw up as much when you're older. Lose weight while you're young."

I sag here and there, but at least I feel young. The good news is I lost weight at age forty-seven, meaning anyone can do it.

This has been my third most meaningful life-changing moment. The first occurred when I became a follower of Jesus Christ. The second came when I married Donna. So the third spot has some gravity. Losing 132 pounds is one of the biggest life-changing events a person could claim.

Mark was right when he said I was on my way to dying early and digging my grave with a fork. Unless I get hit by a bus or die in a plane crash I've probably added ten to fifteen years to my life. That's huge. I haven't added dire, pitiful days and years but good days and years. Healthy, active, productive days and years.

Abundant life has nothing to do with huge portion sizes. In all things, it helps to be content with what God has for us.

All kidding aside, I do ask one favor. I look at how far I've come and cast a hopeful eye at what is ahead. I'm excited and scared at the same time. I trust Jesus but don't trust myself fully. Not yet. I need all the help I can get.

Pray for me.

Acknowledgements

To Tim Luke for working to bring this vision to the printed page. There is no way I could have done this without him. Not only a great writer but a great friend.

To Jason Chatraw and Ampelon Publishing for believing in this project and for all his hard work to get it to the world. Also to Jennifer Wolf—her excellent editing skills make me sound much smarter than I really am.

To my personal weight loss coaches at QWLCA: Tina Couch, Amanda Littlefield, Diann Roberts, and Erica Taylor. These ladies were the best and kept me in line. It's always good to have accountability partners. It didn't hurt that they loved to laugh and have fun, too.

To Billy Lord and Mark Lowry, two of my best friends. They both observed firsthand my journey to heavy city and the return trip to where I am today. I thank them both for being true, sometimes brutally honest, friends.

To my pastor Tim Dowdy and my entire church family at Eagle's Landing First Baptist Church for being there and feeding me all the good spiritual food.

And finally, to my wonderful wife Donna for walking side by side with me during this journey. Most of my humor comes after fighting with her! She loves it. It pays the bills.

About the Author

Scott Davis is a comedian, singer and entertainer. He received Christ at the age of sixteen on July 10, 1979. He graduated from Liberty University where he attended on a full scholarship for traveling with the Light Singers. While working toward his degree in cross-cultural studies, Scott traveled across the U.S. and to ten foreign countries.

Scott's ministry has continued in the U.S. and abroad since his graduation in 1984. He has appeared on Mark Lowry's videos and has written comedy for Mark while under contract with Word Records. For a year, Scott appeared weekly on the national television show, "The Mark & Kathy Show," with Mark Lowry and Kathy Troccoli. Along with his weekly appearances, he has been a guest on numerous religious and secular radio and television broadcasts, including an appearance with comedian Dennis Swanberg on "Swan's Place."

Today, Scott conducts "GET REAL" national conferences with the nation's top speakers and musicians. He also presents music and comedy concert events.

To connect with Scott, visit his website at www.ScottDavis.com.

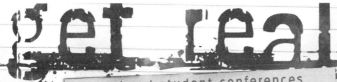

national student conferences

Spiritual Emphasis Conferences for Christian Schools.

These One and Two Day conference events feature the nation's top speakers, musicians, artists, authors, and educators and are uniquely designed to meet the spiritual needs of Christian school students.

During these conferences, students learn to Get Real with themselves, others, and God.

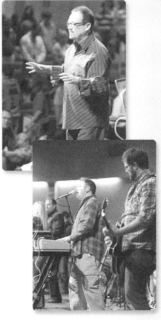

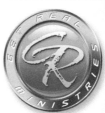

For more information:
www.GetRealNow.us
1-800-356-4963